THE Fl

THE FIFTH SEASON

What it is, how it affects you and how to use those effects
for your health and happiness

Debbie Jolly, M.Ac., L.Ac.
debbiejolly.com

Blazing Valley Press, Sacramento, California

WBLAZING VALLEY PRESS
3560 J Street, Suite 5
Sacramento, CA 95816
916.452-5995

Library of Congress Control Number: 2011916329

ISBN 978-0-9840348-0-2

Printed and bound by All-American Printing, Petaluma,
California.

CAUTIONARY NOTE: The information in this book,
nutritional and otherwise, is in no way intended as a substitute
for counseling with your Medical Doctor.

Table of Contents

✶ Acknowledgements ✶

It's so tempting - and often, in human terms, thrilling! - to think that you're doing something all by yourself. This is especially true when it comes to writing, when you're up there alone in the front bedroom, hunched over your Mac with only the sound of the neighbor's leaf-blower to keep you company; at these times, it does seem that you are doing It all by yourself. But the truth is that each life is the intersection of many different lives.

I want to acknowledge the interest, encouragement and thoughtful feedback of the many wonderful people who oh-so-generously gave of their time and attention to both the birthing and the publishing of this book:

My husband Robert who does many, many things excellently, not the least of which are Being There for me and Giving Good Advice; Regina, Photographer Extraordinaire, who made me look fabulous and helped me with the cover design; the wise and brilliant Jennifer and SuZ who meticulously proofread the final draft, gave me many insights into the book's impact and sprinkled me with magical fairy dust: Elizabeth, the artist with eyes that see so much it's almost scary, who carefully read it and then oh-so-beautifully wrote about it; Walter whose teachings about the world of energy resonate within these pages; Mark, who unhesitatingly gave me the benefit of his own experience as an author and publisher; Sam, who freely offered his technical expertise; Sara, woman of too many talents, who helped me bring the book cover to life; and the warmhearted, giving and amazing clients who gave feedback and advice on the back cover design; encouraged me to publish it in different versions (i.e., eBook and sound recording); and who, miracle of miracles, insisted on paying for that first, spiral-bound "edition" that I had in my waiting room.

I want to thank all of these people for believing in me and for not being shy about showing it.

Finally, I want to thank Bob Duggan, Dianne Connelly, Barbara Ellrich and all my teachers at Tai-Sophia for their vision, their ability to inspire and for a relevant, elevating educational experience. Thanks also to the very sweet and helpful customer service man at Bowker and to Deni and Andrea at All-American who calmly answered a great number of anxious questions about coatings and paper weights and ink colors and shipping times and pdf files and .....

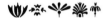

To the spirit of helpfulness, this book is dedicated.

⚕ Chapter One ⚕

The world looks different to me than it does to most people. You see, I'm an acupuncturist. Now, some of you will find this intriguing, while others will probably find themselves unable to get past the idea of needles. After all - *needles???* How in the world are *needles* going to help you feel better? Having been at both ends of the reaction spectrum myself, I can certainly understand both the fascination and the bewilderment; but after close to two decades of making my living as an acupuncturist, <u>my</u> view of what I do is this: Interesting, intelligent, charming people come in and tell me all about themselves. They tell me about their surgeries and their asthma, their back pain and their heartache; they tell me about their childhoods, some of which are wonderful and some absolutely not-wonderful; they tell me about their dreams and their hopes, their despair and their depression, the broken places and the places inside them that aren't. And, from all of this, I try to see one thing: their energy, their life force. I try to see all the different kinds of energy that go to make up the unique beings that they are, how these different kinds of energy are interacting with each other and with the world around them, and, finally, what I can do to help them.

Over the twenty-five years that I've practiced classical acupuncture, I've learned a great deal about what I call energy, what the Chinese call *qi*, what Ayurveda calls *prana*, and what others call 'life force'. I've learned how to recognize the different kinds of energy as they show themselves to me, as they speak to me both from within my clients and from the world around me, from nature. The whole universe is basically a limitless blob of energy and everything in it - every thought, every emotion, every color, every sound, every smell, every object, everything - is an expression of this energy, this Great Oneness. Everything is connected to everything else and there are no barriers.

The seasons, like everything else, are also expressions of energy. They affect us in many ways and at all four levels of our being - the physical, the emotional, the mental, and the spiritual - yet we're often completely unaware of these effects. From the viewpoint of classical acupuncture, the seasonal influences are very specific and understanding them and dealing with them very important to our well-being. So, in 1997, I started writing and distributing a series of newsletters to my clients called *The Point* in which I talked about the nature of each season, how it affects us, what those effects might look like, and how to use these effects for our own benefit. This book is the child of those newsletters.

I had several goals in writing *The Point*: First of all, seasonal effects can often be quite dramatic, and so understanding them can make your life both easier and better. In fact, many of us (just like myself before I became an acupuncturist and I began to think about this kind of thing almost constantly) don't even realize just how much we're affected by the seasonal changes, and in what ways. For instance, down through the years, it's been a normal occurrence to have clients come in during the wintertime complaining of tiredness, a lack of energy, and an inability to get things done. But very few of these poor tired people realized that what they were feeling was a direct result of winter itself. They just thought that there was something wrong with them - that they were either lazy or in the throes of some horrible disease process which had no other symptoms besides exhaustion. They didn't realize that their lack of *oomph* was a natural occurrence, that we all have less energy during wintertime because it's the time of year when the big stream of energy which is constantly flowing into us from the planet narrows down to a trickle. Our planet has its own piece of the big blob of universal energy which ebbs and flows throughout the year, reaching its lowest ebb during wintertime. So, when winter hits our part of the globe, there's a lot less energy available to us and this results in the fact that *we* have less energy. Understanding this - that there was nothing wrong with them, that they were not lazy, worthless slobs but people in the icy grip of winter - helped these clients feel better physically, mentally, emotionally, and even spiritually. Understanding that what they were feeling was normal, natural, and expected went a long way toward improving the quality of their lives, their health, and their sanity.

Secondly, understanding the seasons can help us understand ourselves. Existence as a sentient being is a rich and wonderful thing because there are so many perspectives from which to view it: There's the scientific perspective, the western medical one, the spiritual perspective, the perspectives of psychology and psychotherapy, the family perspective, the individual one, the cultural, the religious, the political, the sexual - the list goes on *ad infinitum,* and the energy perspective is just another way of perceiving the self and its relationship to the world around us. Learning about the seasons is an excellent way to learn about energy - and, therefore, ourselves - because the seasons are expressions of certain types of energy and they're right there, staring us in the face all the time. Looking at things from the viewpoint of energy can be extremely helpful because it's a world without limitations or boundaries. In the world of energy, the body, the mind, the spirit, and the emotions do not exist separate from each other but as different voices of the same whole; and so what goes on in one part of your being must necessarily - and does - affect its other parts. Thus, your asthma, your eczema, your lack of inspiration, your shoulder pain, the fact that your sock drawer is organized according to color, your ability to give guidance to others, and your grief over the loss of your grandmother are all interrelated, intertwined aspects of the self that you call "I", interacting with each other and affecting each other.

But energy is a door that swings both ways. So, if energy doesn't stop at our skins and everything has an effect upon us, it stands to reason that what we do and who we are has an effect upon everything and everyone else. In other words, the world affects us but we also affect it. Yes, each of us is but the tiniest of droplets in the huge swirling soup of energy that we call the universe, but we are *part* of it, not apart from it. Thus, when we work to heal ourselves by having more compassion for the multifaceted cast of characters inside of us, aren't we having the same effect upon the world? When we work to have more inner peace, aren't we also increasing the level of peace on the planet? In the realm of energy, everything's an ecology: Just as the body, the mind, the spirit, and the emotions are basically different expressions or flavors of the oneness inside of us, everything which lives on the planet, from the rocks to the air to the soil to the animals to the plants to the water to the people, are just different voices of the big blob of universal energy, all living the same life, all singing the same song.

The Five Elements 🪷

Energy is limitless. The human consciousness, on the other hand, is based upon the idea of limitation, the idea that "I stop at my skin.". Over the millennia, systems have been created to make this limitlessness, this blob of universal energy, and, therefore, life itself understandable to the human consciousness; and the system which I use is called the Five Elements. Born in India many millennia ago, the Five Elements found its way to China about five thousand years ago, where it became the basis for classical acupuncture, the art of healing people, and *feng shui* or Chinese geomancy, the art of healing environments.

Five Element philosophy states that all energy can be classified into five very distinct types or flavors of energy which we know on planet Earth as water, wood, fire, earth, and metal. Each of the elements has a very distinct character or personality. For instance, the water element is cold, blue, and contracted, while the fire element is hot, red, and expansive. Each of the elements has many, many expressions such as a season, a time of day, a color, a sound, an emotion, a smell, a spirit, parts of the body, powers, etc.. As an example, the seasonal expression of the water element is winter, while the seasonal expression of the fire element is summer. But the most important thing to remember is the *energy comes first*. In other words, before there can be cold, there exists the *energy* of cold. Before blue can exist, the *energy* that we call blue has to exist. We have winter because it's the time of year when this type of cold, blue, contracted energy is most prevalent. We have summer because it's the time of year when the hot, red, expansive energy of the fire element reigns supreme.

The Five Elements are a way of being able to *see* energy; for, as a system, the Five Elements asks us to see the oceans and the trees and the fires and the fields and the gemstones within us. Because energy doesn't stop at our skins, the very same energy which created the oceans and the rivers - the energy of the water element - is within us; and so we, too, possess the same ability to be powerful, tranquil, and liquid that we feel when we stand on the shore and watch the waves roll in. The same energy which created the diamond and gave it its sparkle, its brilliance - the energy of the metal element - is there within us; and so that same sparkle, that same brilliance, that same energy of worth and riches and richness dwells within us as well. The same energy which expresses itself as the sun, its warmth and its power to illuminate - the energy of the fire element - is within us, revealing itself in that same ability to shine, to give off warmth, and to light up the world. The same energy which allows a tiny, defenseless seedling to burst through the crusty soil - the energy of the wood element - is within us, ready for any challenge, ready to start over again and create the world anew. And the same energy which expresses itself as the ground, the soil beneath our feet, as well as this home we call planet Earth - the energy of the earth element - is also within us, supporting us, feeding us, nurturing us so that we can feed and support and nurture not just ourselves, but anyone else that we want to gather to our breast and take care of.

The elements are there, talking to us all the time. The wonderful thing about the Five Elements as a system is that, on some level, we already know everything there is to know about water, wood, fire, earth, and metal because we have daily experience of them, whether it's through turning on the tap in order to wash the dishes or in stopping to watch the river flow by, unstoppable, willful, and powerful, on its way to the ocean. The wonderful thing about the seasons is that they're another voice of the elements, another way into ourselves and the world within us, and another way out of ourselves into the world around us, the world in which we live and of which we are inextricably a part.

How To Use This Book ❀

Nothing that we experience has just one cause. Everything that we experience at any given moment - whether it's pain in the elbow or depression or cancer - is actually the intersection of the many, many different things which are going on inside of us and outside of us simultaneously. At any single point in time, we're being acted upon by a multitude of influences; the seasonal effects are one of these and their effects can be quite significant and overarching. We usually can't control what's going on in our exterior landscape, but we *can* adjust our interior one by changing how we see things, and that's where *The Fifth Season* comes in.

What originally started out as a book about all five seasons has become a book about one: late summer, also known as "Indian Summer". While summer starts right around June 21, the summer solstice, it only lasts for seven weeks, after which late summer, the time of decrease and sweetness and heaviness and falling-apart, begins. While late summer shares some of summer's characteristics and thus may *seem* like summer (warm days that are still fairly long.), energetically it's as different as yellow is from red, as sympathy is from joy, as heavy is to light, and as sweet is to bitter.

If you have to pick only one of the five seasons to write about, late summer is probably the best choice. First of all, it's said that, because the energy of late summer is that of a big mixing bowl that accepts everything and leaves nothing out, all the other seasons are actually present within it. Secondly, late summer is about the body and the care of the body. Thirdly, you could just as easily call it the mother element, because that's what it is: the energy of home and mother and caring for and needs and neediness and satisfaction and sensuality. So, a book about late summer is at the same time a book about caring for yourself.

Late summer, which lasts from about the end of the first week of August until the fall equinox, is the time when the earth element reigns supreme; so during this season, all of its many expressions (also known as 'correspondences') are much more easily seen and felt. Reading the book and performing the Home Treatment suggestions will be a little different during this time; but because the energy of the earth element is present all the time, you would get just as much out of my book at the other times of year, albeit in a slightly different way.

The Story is meant to evoke the energetic essence of the season and how it makes us feel. The "Home Treatment" section gives suggestions for what you can do to use the season's positive effects for your benefit and healing while diminishing what are seen as negative ones. The poem and the essay in "The Bigger Picture" offer other vantage points from which to understand the particular energy of the season and its effect.

Of course, you don't need to be plagued by pesky symptoms in order to use or enjoy this book. You can use it as a window from which to see the world and yourself in a new way, a more expanded way, a way which offers you more resources and, ultimately, more hope. *The Fifth Season* was written to help you, the reader, see yourself and your life from the perspective of energy and thus, from the perspective of interconnectedness. And the ability to see yourself in this way is a precious one, for it's something which can help you have more happiness, more fulfillment, and more trust in yourself.

The Fifth Season was also written to entertain you. A client once said to me, "I come for the show but I stay for the acupuncture". Entertainment tends to be regarded as frivolous and superficial; but to me, healing and entertainment have a lot in common, for both of them have the ability to expand us, to help us, to transform us, and to bring us joy. So, if you get nothing else from this book but an entertaining read, I'll feel that I've accomplished my goal. If, in reading this book, you are able to see yourself or the world in an expanded way, even if it's just for a moment, I'll feel that I've accomplished what I set out to do. Life on planet Earth is a wild, colorful, crazy ride, terrifying and gratifying in equal measure; and if I can help by increasing your level of joy while decreasing your level of misery, in any way or on any level, I'll be a happy woman.

I hope that you enjoy my book. 🎭🎭

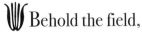 Behold the field,
>   the bosom of the Earth.
>   Behold this Great Horizontal,
>   this Heavenly Pivot,
>   this home to which we,
>   severally wounded, winded,
>   stripped of will, hope,
>   fatigued in body, with mind confus*ed*
>   and spirit broken,
>   return. 〰

A Story about Late Summer

It's a morning in late August, and you're sitting outside on your patio taking a break. The sun is warm and soft on your skin, and the air is dense and full of moisture. All around you, bees drone as they float from flower to flower, steady in their concentration and busy in their task. Above the murmur of the bees is the sound of the birds talking to each other, a relaxed conversation that starts and stops, starts and stops. The murmur of the bees and the chatter of the birds are two different and distinct types of sounds, two different kinds of music which fit together like a symphony, a song of late summer.

The perfume of flowers and recently-cut grass comes to you in waves and you inhale, filling your lungs with the smell of sweetness and nourishment. There's a certain color that you associate with this time of year, a pale golden-yellow, and you notice that there's a lot of it in the area right around you. The garden, overgrown and bursting at the seams, is in serious need of some weeding and pruning, and, looking around yourself for a diversion, you notice some grapes growing a few inches from you. Leaning as far as you can out of your chair without actually having to get up, you pick one and eat it. Your taste buds do a little dance of happiness. You pick and eat another one and your eyes close with pleasure. Sighing, you relax more deeply into your chair, laughing at the intense heaviness of body and the weariness that you feel. After all, all you did was sweep your tiny little porch -- and only half of it at that.

But the tiredness and the weariness are actually pleasant, and your body feels good -- or maybe you just feel good in your body. It's so nice out here that soon you stop wondering about anything. Thoughts slip out of your mind and for a moment or two there's nothing but the movement of the bees, the sounds of the birds, the caress of the wind, the warmth of the sun, and the way that the air is full of scent and moisture. Sitting there in your back yard on this morning in late summer, you're starting to feel so, well, mellow that even the sight of weeds growing out of control can't do anything to ruin the moment for you. After all, it's just another sign of Earth's abundance, just another message from the planet that it can support more life than you'd ever thought possible. So, even with the rest of the patio beckoning, you give yourself over to the moment and let yourself sit there a little while longer, taking all of this in and letting it lull and comfort you. You feel the weight of your body against the chair. You feel how the chair is holding you in all your contentedness and your tiredness, and you slouch down into it even more. Your head falls back onto the headrest and you watch little clouds drifting overhead, lazy like you. Your legs feel heavy, oh so heavy, and you lift them up onto the bench in front of you. And then you let yourself absorb the feel and the rhythms of your back yard in late summer, this gentle, swaying universe of music and movement.

Watching the bees drag their heavy little bodies through the equally heavy air, you realize that there's something familiar about the way they're acting, about the way they laboriously penetrate each flower, intent only upon their task and oblivious to the beauty around them. You look around you. Suddenly you feel enveloped by everything all at once: the abundance and strength of the earth, the force of green things growing way past their prime, the nourishment and the sweetness, the warmth and the laziness, the murmurings and the toil, the gentleness and the generosity of the pale yellow morning. And for a second, all of these things exist together as one; for a moment, the sights, the sounds, the smells, and the feelings have all coalesced into one single thing. You can't even say what it is but it's definitely there, forming a circle around you and somehow you're part of it, this oneness of sensation and nature and time. And then from out of this oneness, this force of sweetness and strength, the thought of suffering arises. You think of all those who have suffered or are suffering right now, the thousands or millions for whom life is a hard bed and an empty bowl. It's as though they're there with you, standing under the August sun, with eyes that have seen too much and hands which have held too little, a wall of sorrow released from the circle around you. They are your brothers and your sisters, your kith and your kin, and though you know you'll never be able to help them, part of you reaches out to them.

All at once, it's cooler and the garden deepens in shadow. The sun has gone behind a cloud. You look over at the unswept patio, and it seems to be calling to you. You realize that the sorrow in your gut is existing side-by-side with the earlier feelings of pleasure and satisfaction. It seems incomprehensible that one hasn't obliterated the other, but, after all, what do you know? What do you really know -- about anything? The now-muted light, the shadows in the garden make it look both mysterious and inviting, full of things that you can only guess at: fairies, nymphs, giant slugs eating your roses. The soil beneath your feet, the dark rich earth which you tilled in the springtime and which grew peaches and strawberries in summer, is also growing a huge crop of weeds. But it doesn't matter. Abundance is all around you. The bosom of mother Earth is supporting you, holding you up. Hauling yourself to your feet once more, you pick up your broom and go back to work. ❀ ❀ ❀

⚹ Chapter Two ⚹
Everything you need and plenty of it

Wait just a minute, you might be saying to yourself, what's all this about a fifth season? Late *summer*?! Is this a real season or just a continuation of summer itself? Well, dear readers, the answer is, No, late summer *is* a real season; it's the time between the maximum expansion of summer and the return-to-within that is fall. It's the time of year when the energy of the Earth, which came rocketing out in springtime to reach its peak in summer, begins its journey back to the depths, a journey which ends in the long sleep that is winter. So while summer is the time of expansion and light, late summer is the time of decrease and solidity. Late summer is the seasonal expression of the energy of the earth element; and, like the earth beneath our feet which supports us and gives to us a home, the energy of late summer is heavy, hard to move, and subject to the laws of gravity. For in late summer, the intangible weightlessness of summer has been converted into something tangible and weighty; and as the energy of the planet starts to wane and move downward, we feel a sense of heaviness in ourselves and in the world around us.

Late summer is a time of roundness, ripeness, and sweetness. The weather, while still hot, is just a bit cooler and slightly humid. The days are markedly shorter, there's a heaviness to the air, and everything seems to be moving more slowly. The fruits which reached maximum size during the summer now hang heavy on the vine, juicy and ripe and ready for picking. The fields and gardens are filled with the low murmur of insect life as a myriad butterflies and bees float from flower to flower, gathering sustenance in the face of the approaching winter. Everything seems a little frayed around the edges and just a bit past its prime, ready either for the harvest or for the housecleaning of fall. It's the time of abundance, the time when we can most clearly see that the Earth is our mother, our support, and our lunch box. For everywhere we look, we see evidence of her generosity, from the legions of grasshoppers in our fields that explode with every step we take, to the overgrowth of grasses and weeds in our gardens, to the orchards bursting with pears that threaten to succumb to the pull of gravity if not picked. It's a golden time, a time of mellowness and satisfaction, a time when the energies of sensuality and plenty prevail. And yet it's also a time of sorrow. For, as the days shorten and we begin the descent toward the inevitable, waiting depths of winter, our mood, like the light, like the energy of the Earth, like our own level of energy, begins to wane as well; and as our focus is pulled from the lightfilled peaks of summer back downward toward the Earth, the contentment that we feel is tinged with a slight melancholy, a recognition that Earth's abundance comes hand in hand with what to our human minds is a price.

This is the time of year when things ripen. The process of ripening is a series of steps by which larger, more complex starch molecules are broken down into simpler molecules of sugar; thus ripening is the process by which something literally falls apart. Energy doesn't stop at our skins, and so during late summer this process of ripening is happening within us as well. Thus, as the fruits and vegetables in our gardens ripen and their starch molecules break down and fall apart, it can feel to us as though we -- and our lives -- are falling apart as well. And, in a way, our lives *are* falling apart. Late summer is a time of transition; it's the bridge which allows us to cross over from the red-hot excitement of summer into the cool introspection of fall. These two seasons are very different from each other, and the ride from one to the next would be a bumpy one indeed if it were not for the transitional nature of late summer. And this is where ripening comes in. Ripening allows the joyful energy of summer to break down into its component parts so that it can eventually be transformed into the letting-go of fall. And so the ripening of our lives -- the process by which our lives break down into their component parts -- is a necessary part of the transition we make from summer to fall, from joy to grief, from being outwardly-focussed to inwardly-, from celebration to inspiration. The energy of ripening brings sweetness to our lives, but it can also make them feel disjointed and out of kilter. But we have help. For this is also the time of year when the energy of mother and mothering is strongest, and therefore the time of year when it's easiest to connect with our own ability to be the mother and supportive presence to ourselves. The warm, nurturing energy of late summer shows us how to be the mother who is always there for us, the mother who cares for us and takes care of us, the mother who holds us and listens to our needs and tries to fill them. And so, as we make the shift from summer to fall and the lighthearted energy of celebration begins to ripen and disintegrate, the solid, tangible energy of this time of year is, like the supportive bosom of mother Earth itself, something which allows us to make this transition in one piece.

One of the expressions of the earth element, and thus of late summer itself, is the bowl. The bowl is a very female energy: a receptive form whose rounded shape allows it to hold things. Like the Earth beneath our feet, which accepts all that falls onto it and gives to it a home, the bowl provides a place for each and every item which is put into it, no matter how different these things are from one another. It is said that, in the seasonal cycle, late summer is the bowl. For during late summer, all the seasons are present. The light of summer, the stillness of winter, the vision of springtime, and the inspiration of fall all have a place within the warm, accepting embrace of late summer. The bowl-like energy of late summer thus gives us a receptacle for holding and accepting the many pieces of our lives. To integrate is to unify, and thus create a oneness from, disparate elements. When we make a cake, for instance, we take ingredients which are chemically and physically quite different from each other -- eggs, flour, vanilla, honey, baking powder, milk, oil, nuts, and salt -- and put all of them into a mixing bowl. Some of the ingredients are from animal sources, some are from plant sources, and some are from mineral sources; some are sweet, some are salty, some are bitter, some are neutral; some are watery, some are dry, and some are oily. Yet, within the rounded confines of the mixing bowl, all of these items have a place, all of them are accepted, and all of them belong. Within the rounded confines of the mixing bowl, the animal resides next to the vegetable and the sweet next to the salty. Within the rounded confines of the mixing bowl, all of these items are accepted, held, and finally mixed together to create one single thing: cake batter. And so as the party lights of summer fade and we look ahead to fall, the bowl-like nature of this time of year gives us a way to take all that happened in the months or years before -- the many events, impressions, thoughts, facts, emotions, and physical changes -- and to create a oneness from it. The integrating, unifying energy of late summer helps us make a place where the happy and the sad, the bitter and the sweet, the failures and the successes can come together and form a unity.

Late summer is the time of year when we digest our lives. Digestion is a process, and the first part of this process is to take what we have and break it down into smaller, more understandable pieces. The second part of the process is to take these pieces and use them to create something which will nourish us. The first power of late summer, then, the power to take something apart and mull it over, gives us a way to understand ourselves, our lives, and our world. The second power of late summer, the power to take these bits and pieces and to create something new with them, gives us a way to transform the past and the present into the future. On a physical level, then, digestion is the process by which we transform the food we eat into flesh. On a mental level, it's the process by which we transform facts, sensory impressions, and the ideas of others into our own thoughts and ideas. Sitting in the gentle, diminished light of late summer, cradled and supported by the energy of the Earth, we have the chance to dismantle all that came before and consider the pieces. And then, bolstered by the limitless ability of the Earth to support and feed us, we have the opportunity to take these pieces and transform them into something which will nourish our bodies, our minds, our emotions, and our spirits in the coming months and years.

Each element, and thus each season, has a direction which corresponds to it. Winter's direction is north, the direction of least sun; spring's direction is east, the direction of the rising sun; the direction of summer is south, the direction of greatest and midday sun; while the direction of autumn is west, the direction of the setting sun. But the direction of late summer is center, and this is the time of year when the energy pulls our focus away from our edges and in toward our middles. This helps us as we try to digest our lives because, in Chinese medicine, the middle of the body is where all of our processing and transformation -- in other words, all of our digestion -- takes place. But the centering aspect of late summer helps us with the digestive process in yet another way. For, as our attention is pulled away from our borders and in toward the centers of who we are, we have less of an inclination to continue taking in new things and more of an inclination to process what we've already consumed. The ability to focus on the center of who we are -- that is, to center ourselves -- and to digest what we have right now gives us a chance to be with ourselves in a way that grounds us before the steep downhill slide of fall carries us away into the future.

The energy of late summer is the energy of the physical, the energy of the tangible, the energy of that which we can see and hear and smell and touch; and, thus late summer is the time of the body and its needs. As human beings, we tend to feel that who we are is defined by our bodies because they are the supreme expressions of our individuality. But even though our bodies are so important to us, we often find it hard or even impossible to give them what they need when they need it. The season of late summer gives us a chance to understand the realities of our bodies, and to hear what they need and give this to them. But because it's the time of year when it's easiest to understand our physical form, it's also the time of year when the vulnerability of that physical form is most obvious to us as well. Our bodies are the expressions of our own individual drops of universal energy, yet the rules which govern them are very different from those which govern energy. For one thing, energy is indestructible and limitless, while our bodies are not. The body is fragile and vulnerable to a host of forces, many of which are beyond our control. And so, as the energy of the planet begins to decrease and fall away and the fragility of the body becomes more evident, late summer can be a time of great insecurity. But it can also be a time of great pleasure as well. For during late summer, the energy of sensuality is at its peak, and so our bodies, which can be sources of great anxiety, can also be sources of great pleasure as well. Having a body puts us in a position which is uniquely precarious, but it also allows us to have pleasures that we couldn't experience without them. The sweet, mellow, body-centered energy of late summer reminds us that to be human and have a body is both an uncertain reality and a vastly rewarding one.

Late summer, the seasonal expression of the earth element, is the time to look inward to find the mother inside of us. It's the time when the Earth cradles us with her unstinting generosity, the time when we look to the planet to learn how best to care for ourselves and to become for ourselves the mother who is always there for us when we call out in the night, the constant presence who listens for our voice and who cares about us, the kind hand that soothes the worried brow, the soft and melodious voice that sings to us a song of abundance, the substantial presence which calms our fears and rocks us gently, oh so gently as she spins us on her axis, sweetly, kindly, holding us, supporting us as we start to fall downward, downward, downward back toward the darkness of winter. ❀ ❀ ❀

Before we continue . . .

As you go on to the Home Treatment section, Dear Reader, please bear in mind that - as I have tried to stress - everyone is unique. Everyone's individual energy systems are unique, everyone's biochemistries and medical histories are unique and this means that everyone's needs are also unique. Before trying any of my suggestions, please consult with your physician. For that's what the following are: suggestions, not prescriptions or rules. Even though they are suggestions born of a quarter-century of experience as a healthcare professional, strongly-held beliefs and lots of thought on my part, they are nonetheless ideas that I am putting forth to you which should be discussed with your doctor first, before putting any of them into practice.

✣ Chapter Three ✣
Home Treatment

The energy of each season offers us both gifts and challenges. Here are some ideas on how to recognize and make use of the gifts of late summer while understanding and minimizing the effects of its challenges.

✿ Sympathy

Let yourself go back to the late summer back yard of the Story of Late Summer. See yourself sitting outside in that back yard. Now imagine that you can feel the warmth of the sun on your body, and the comfort of your body in its chair. All around you, you can see and hear the bees as they drone from flower to flower, heavy with pollen, and their murmurings fill the air in a comforting way. And, as they float and land, float and land, and move up and down, up and down at different times in their slow, heavy way, they seem to be doing a ballet. You watch them rise and fall, rise and fall, energies which are separate but which are all engaged in the same task, and the breeze against your skin is soft and warm. It's such a gentle morning. You inhale and your chest expands with a full, slow breath; you smell the fragrance of flowers and the sweetness of just-mowed grass. You can see that the back yard and the garden are overfilled with flowers and grasses and weeds and that you're surrounded by a lot of a certain color, a soft golden-yellow. As you watch the bees float and land, float and land, a word comes into your consciousness and you hear the word in your head: "Sympathy". You look out at the scene around you. You see the bees move up and down, up and down in the fragrant, heavy air. You watch them rise

and fall, rise and fall, float and land, float and land; and in your head you hear, "Sympathy ....
sympathy ....sympathy .... sympathy" over and over in time with the swaying, lilting rhythm of the late summer world around you.

This is an exercise designed to help you to have a better understanding of sympathy, the emotional expression of the energy of late summer. When we look at the world from the perspective of energy, what we see is that energy comes first and everything else - every object, feeling, emotion, force, color, temperature, movement, sound, everything - is an expression of that energy. By allowing yourself to enter into the back yard and immerse yourself in the energy of late summer, you give yourself the opportunity to understand one of its expressions - the emotion of sympathy - in a more complete way. The word sympathy comes from "syn", which means together, and "pathy", which means to feel. Sympathy is thus the ability to feel with - and therefore to feel for - another. It's the emotional state that a mother has toward her child, an emotion which says to that child, "Yes, I feel for you and I am here with you." Sympathy is thus the emotion which allows us to be open to another and to their needs. Sympathy is often thought of as the state of feeling sorry for someone or something. But sympathy is simply a quality of attention; it's an emotional posture which says, verbally or nonverbally, to someone else, "Yes, I am here with you." And sympathy can come in many forms, from the more gooey and expressive variety ("Oh, you poor thing!") which usually involves holding or touching in order to let the other person know that he or she is not alone and that you're there with him or her, to a type of attentive listening in which no words or actions are involved. Sympathy is thus an emotion in which we extend our awareness and our willingness to "feel together with" another being, human or otherwise. And so, as you see yourself in the pale golden-yellow garden, as you watch the slow waltz of the bees and hear their droning, as you feel the warmth and softness of the air and smell its fragrance, you're allowing yourself to have a fuller understanding of the true nature of the emotion of sympathy from an energy standpoint.

Each of the elemental energies has many, many expressions, which are also called 'correspondences'. The correspondences include a time of day, a time of year, a sound, an emotion, a smell, a color, parts of the body, powers, and abilities, to name just a few. Thus, as above, understanding a particular energy allows us to understand its correspondences. But the reverse is also true, and the correspondences are helpful in understanding the energy of a particular season and how it affects us. Like the tips of icebergs, the correspondences are the visible portions of a much bigger reality. They are a set of clues that allow us to track down - and ultimately understand - a certain type of energy. If the energy of an element is the room, then the correspondences are the doors through which we can enter into that room and the windows through which we can see into it. So, for example, the singing voice; the sweet taste; the spleen and the stomach; the mouth; the color yellow; the fragrant smell; the humid climate; and the season of late summer are all different voices which express a single, larger reality: the energy of the earth element. To us as human beings, the emotions are rich, vivid, sometimes disturbing energies which seem very real and which make our lives seem very real as well. Because of this, emotions are particularly compelling as voices of the elemental energies and exploring them is an excellent way to understand a specific season. Thus, as a way into understanding the energy of late summer, what does sympathy show us? That it's the time of year when our ability to be attentive to others and their needs may deepen. That it's the time of year when our ability to be there for ourselves may deepen. That it's the time of year when our ability to "feel together with" our surroundings - e.g., the natural world - may deepen. Each season offers us its own unique way of experiencing our connection to the world around us and late summer is no exception. Like a mother with her awareness extended out toward her sleeping child and listening for the first cry of need, the emotion of sympathy allows us to extend our attention outward from our centers in order to come into resonance with everyone and everything around us.

So, during this season of nourishment and needs, give yourself the opportunity to see how you are with this emotion. Because this is the time of year when the energy of sympathy is strongest, you might notice something about yourself in relationship to this emotion that you hadn't noticed before. Are you constantly listening outside of yourself to everyone else's needs and deaf to your own? Those of us who do this usually have an excellent idea of what's going on with others and a very poor concept of what's going on inside ourselves. Or is the reverse scenario true for you? Are you continually stuck inside yourself with little or no idea of what's going on with others? Are you able to extend yourself outward in order to understand - on an emotional level - what's going on with someone else? Are you able to give sympathy to others? Sympathy is often a response to the needs and neediness that we perceive in others, and we human beings often have a very, very, very hard time with needs because they scare us. They scare us because they're evidence of the truth of human existence: that we're not self-sufficient; that all of us are dependent upon the world around us and therefore vulnerable to it. And so, faced with the neediness of others, some of us respond not with sympathy but with emotions such as fear or anger. Give yourself a gift. Try to make this a time when you look at your ability to give - and to receive - sympathy from others. Then try to determine what you need to do to make a balance in this regard. Some of us are champion sympathizers but, when the balm of sympathy is extended toward us, we shut down, clam up, or push it away. Often this happens because we have an imbalance in our stomach energy and thus have difficulty taking in what we need. Sometimes we have trouble accepting sympathy from others - or from ourselves - because we interpret sympathy as a judgment of our worth and/or our ability to deal with a certain situation. Sometimes an inability to accept sympathy is a defense to keep what's going on inside of you a secret - from others, but also from yourself. Some of us are excellent at receiving sympathy but have trouble reading others and extending this to them. And some of us respond to the signals that others send out which are actually appeals for sympathy with jokes (well intentioned or otherwise) or barbs, or both, while still others see the need for sympathy as a sign of weakness and then zero in for the kill. An inability to give sympathy often comes from a deep discomfort with the emotions in general; those who are unable to give of themselves in this way tend to view the emotions as a vast wasteland into which no sane, levelheaded person would venture. These people often have very good minds and are able to understand others in a mental, or intellectual, way; but when it comes to being

with others, or with themselves, in an emotional way ....
well, that's a threshold they just can't seem to cross. There
is no right or wrong way of giving or receiving sympathy.
There is no standardized level of "appropriate" sympathy-
giving or -receiving. Each of us has within us many, many,
many different types of energy which are all put together in
a very unique way; and so the relationship that each of us
has to sympathy is unique. Thus, the only person who
knows what your level of sympathy "should" be is you, for
you're the authority, the boss of yourself. No one else can
claim that right.

During these golden days of late summer, try to
approach the whole issue of sympathy with compassion for
yourself and for others. Compassion is simply
acknowledging what's in front of you, staring you in the
face. Thus, for some of us, compassion is finally allowing
yourself to see that what you've been tripping over all these
years is your need for others to give to you - or you to
them. Being human can be a scary thing, and having needs
can be terrifying. The energy of this time of year is one
which makes our own neediness and the neediness of
others glaringly evident to us; but it's also one which says
that there's something which can help take the sting out of
having those needs, and that thing is sympathy. For
sympathy creates a pathway between entities: The party
giving sympathy extends themselves outward and the party
receiving the sympathy opens up in order to take it in.
Therefore, sympathy is one of the roadways through which
we can nourish and take care of each other. As human
beings, we often feel isolated, alone, and lacking enough of
whatever it is that we feel we need. But even though the
human form predisposes us to see our lives as a glass which
is half full, the reality of the universe is that it's a place of

abundant, limitless energy and the giving and receiving of sympathy allows us to experience this abundance on an emotional level. The giving and receiving of sympathy allows us to *feel* that we're not alone; it allows us to feel and to experience, in a very direct way, our connection to each other and to everything else. When we allow ourselves to give or receive sympathy, we give ourselves a chance to see that having needs is not an exercise in helplessness but merely evidence of our connection to the world around us. The making and taking of sympathy is thus just another way of affirming that we're all part of the same oneness and that, from an energy perspective, the universe is something filled to the top and brimming over and that it's a place of safety, not a place of danger. ♪ ♪

❀ Make Your Life Sweet

The sweet taste is a very compelling one. For many of us, it's the taste we long for, especially when life gets complicated, scary, or difficult. And we *should* have sweets in our lives, for sometimes it's the cookie or piece of pumpkin pie or the hot fudge sundae which gives us a reason to keep going when life doesn't seem to be offering us a good enough one to do so. Huge industries have been built up around the sweet taste which every year churn out massive quantities of cookies, bakery goods, candies, and ice cream and ferry them in fleets of trucks to stores where we, the customers, wait openmouthed like hatchlings to be fed. So what is it, exactly, about the sweet taste that so attracts us?

In order to answer that, we need to understand taste from an energy standpoint. Each of the five elements has many expressions, or correspondences, and taste is one of them. The taste which corresponds to the water element, and thus to the season of winter, is the salty taste, the taste of the ocean. In Chinese medicine, salty things have the ability to soften and purge, and these qualities are an expression of winter's ability to dissolve and cleanse. The watery energy of winter allows us to dissolve the past and wash it away, leaving us to face the core of who we are in the ensuing silence and purity. Thus, every time we eat a piece of *sushi* or the anchovies on a pizza or in a caesar salad, what we're getting, along with the iodine and other minerals, is this essence of simplicity and silence. The taste which corresponds to the wood element, and thus to the season of springtime, is the sour taste, the taste of lemons and limes and grapefruit. The sour taste has a contracting, or astringent, effect and this reflects the very nature of springtime itself. For spring is the time of year when the energy allows us to pull in all our flaps and focus forward as we barrel ahead and take a flying leap into the future. Thus, every time we bite into a slice of lemon or eat a piece of grapefruit, what we're getting along with the vitamin C and potassium is a little taste of springtime's arrow of focus. The taste of the fire element, and thus of the season of summer, is the bitter taste, the taste of things that have been burned or scorched. The bitter taste is therefore a smoky distillation of summer itself; for summer is, in its own way, a time of purification, a time when all that is extraneous is burned away by the sun and the heat, and all that's left is the only thing that matters: our relationship to each other. And so, when you drink a cup of coffee, eat a piece of chocolate or a piece of burned toast (yes, some of us like our toast *actually* toasted), you're also feeding yourself a little bit of summer's energy of love and connection. The taste of the metal element, and thus of the season of autumn, is the spicy taste; and in Chinese medicine, the spicy taste has a dispersing or scattering effect. Once again, this is an expression of the essence of autumn; for autumn is the time of year when the energy of the planet is moving back down toward the earth, urging us to clean out our internal and external closets and let go of what no longer serves us. But fall is also the time of year when the energy of the planet is moving up toward the heavens and pulling our focus with it, asking us to determine what adds a sense of richness and quality to our lives. And so, every time we take a bite of curry or a bite of chicken baked with oregano and basil, we bring this energy of richness, meaning, and value into ourselves. For within the spicy taste lives the essence of autumn, that time when the heavenly and the earthly walk hand in hand.

The taste which corresponds to the earth element, and thus to the season of late summer, is the sweet taste, and the sweet taste is a harmonizing and strengthening one. Once again, this is an expression of the essence of late summer, for late summer is the time of year when all the seasons are present in equal measure, when everything is accepted and nothing is left out. It's the time of year when the gentleness and the warmth make it possible to see, and to accept, the many different aspects which live inside of us and to make peace with the fact that we, like life itself, are many-splendored things. It's also the time of year when a certain kind of strength, the strength which comes from being supported, is most available to us. For, every minute of every day, we experience the support of the Earth; every minute of every day, we derive strength from her. And, in the soft, yellow light of late summer, we can see our planet for what she is: a mighty chunk of rock hurtling through space, carrying trillions and gillions of beings and non-beings on her back, feeding us and giving all of us a home. Therefore, every time we take a bite of a hot fudge sundae or a cookie or taste a piece of pie, we're bringing this energy of agreement and support, this music of harmony and might into every drop of our being.

Unfortunately, the actual consumption of sweets is something which has created discord instead of harmony. It's a subject riddled with controversy - Are sweets good for us? Is refined sugar actually a gift from Satan? - and with questions to which there are no easy answers. The reality is that it's important to have an experience of life which tells us that it's sweet: It's vital to our health and it's indispensable to our willingness to keep going forward; and eating sweets gives us a very good way of doing this. The problem is that it's often hard, or impossible, for some of us to have a balance when it comes to eating sweets. What is balance? you may ask. Balance is the ability to experience something without getting stuck in it. Let's look at the world of emotions for further explanation. According to Chinese medicine, emotional health (i.e., balance) has three parts: (1) the ability to experience each of the five emotions; (2) the ability to experience, or go into, a particular emotion in a way that matches the situation; and (3) the ability to get out of that emotion when we feel complete with it, and to go on. The same guidelines apply to the world of tastes, and balance here means being able to visit each of the five tastes without being kidnapped and held hostage by one of them. This is more difficult for some of us than for others when it comes to sweets. Many people have a very hard time saying 'no' to the call of the Siren of Sweetness in the first place; and then, once they've answered, it's even harder for them to stop answering, and soon the sweet taste begins to rule their lives. Since this is the time of year when the energy of sweetness is at its peak, the ways in which sweets affect us are most obvious; so we have help in understanding ourselves and making changes. Here, then, are a few ideas which may help bring a little balance to this issue.

Use refined sweeteners such as granulated sugar, confectioner's sugar, corn syrup, and brown sugar sparingly. It's been said that "sugar is sugar is sugar", that, in other words, there's no difference between eating refined sugar and more "natural" forms of sugar such as honey, molasses, or maple syrup. My own opinion - which may not be in tune with that of nutritional science - is that refined sugar is something best taken in small quantities. Because it's refined, it has no nutritional value except for sucrose, a chemical compound in which a molecule of glucose is linked to a molecule of fructose. All the trace minerals and vitamins of the sugar beet or sugar cane have been stripped away and what we have left is something which is, to my mind at least, remarkably similar to a drug. For, taken in large enough quantities, the result of eating refined sugar is that a lot of pure glucose (sugar) is released into the bloodstream all at once, giving us that nice sugar high. Sometimes, of course, this drug-like effect is exactly what we're after. And, while drugs are perfectly valid substances which add a great deal to our lives, they're not foods. Foods nourish, while drugs are used to affect ourselves in very specific ways. For example, we use coffee and tea to sharpen mental acuity and overcome fatigue, while erythromycin is used to fight infection and codeine is used to kill pain. Thus, refined sugar doesn't really have the ability to add anything to your life nutritionally; and so, when eating refined sweeteners, try to determine whether you're after nourishment or whether you're trying to affect yourself in a different way.

Let me offer something which you may find helpful - my Rule of Thumb: Try to minimize your consumption of refined foods. They have been stripped of many, if not all, of their attendant nutrients and micro-nutrients, such as minerals and vitamins. Many claim that the quantities in which these nutrients appear in unrefined sweeteners are much too small to add anything of value to our diet; however, in light of the fact that nutritional science is in a state of constant change, it's probably best to keep an open mind and not discount the presence of these nutritional gems in any quantity. And then there's the Caveperson Factor. Refined foods were first available during the Industrial Revolution, which means that they've only been around for about 150 years, while the species to which we belong, *Homo sapiens sapiens* has been around for about 40,000. Thus our bodies are probably set up to handle the type of nutrition which was available many millennia ago, and the more our diet resembles that of a caveperson, the better. For, while our minds may be in the twenty-first century, in many ways our bodies are not. ✓

Mitigate the effect of refined sweeteners. Refined carbohydrates like table sugar and white flour are metabolized more quickly than whole grains and unrefined sweeteners because fewer steps are needed by the body to break them down into glucose (sugar). White flour, like other refined grains, has been processed so that the germ, which is rich in vitamin E and other nutrients, and the indigestible bran have been removed. Thus, white flour can convert to its component sugars more quickly than whole grains can. Eating cookies or cakes made with white flour *and* refined sugar is in some ways like throwing a piece of very, very dry wood on a fire: the fire is very hot and hard to control, the wood burns too quickly, and you only have heat and light for a short time. This is especially problematic for those who are sensitive to changes in their blood sugar because it affects the way they feel on a physical level in a noticeable, and sometimes dramatic, way.

You can offset the effect of refined sugars by packaging them differently. In other words, if you like to bake, try using refined sweeteners together with whole grains to make cookies, cakes, and pastries. Or try using whole and refined grains or flours together. Chocolate chip cookies using 2/3 whole wheat and 1/3 white flour are incredibly delicious, and pear pie made with a whole-wheat crust is even better. Pumpkin pie is so much more yummy in a crust made of brown rice flour and almond oil. Eating whole foods gives you the type of fire which burns more slowly and evenly, and which gives off heat and light (i.e., energy) for a longer period of time. And since whole grains are naturally sweeter than refined flours, less sugar is needed to sweeten them; plus, they often have a wonderful flavor of their own. Whole grains are also much more nutritious than their refined cousins, and so using them in your baking allows you to do something which we don't usually associate with the consumption of goodies: nourish yourself. If you don't like to bake, it's possible to find these products in natural foods stores and in the natural foods sections in supermarkets. In fact, there's a whole world of sweets made with unrefined or less-refined ingredients just waiting to be discovered, including frozen desserts made from soy (which tastes a lot like ice cream) and brown rice (which doesn't but which is incredibly good anyway); and the all-important chocolate, which comes sweetened with fruit juice or with cane syrup. In fact, chocolate has so much to offer us nutritionally that it's worth your while to seek out the type made with unrefined and less-refined sugars; for, in addition to nourishment, some of the most delicious chocolate on the market these days is sweetened this way.

Carbohydrates are metabolized more quickly than fats or proteins. Thus, another good way to mitigate the effects of refined sweeteners is to eat them with fats and proteins. Doing this allows the simple sugars to enter the bloodstream more slowly. So, in other words, have a piece or three of candy or a brownie at the end of a meal. The negative effects of refined sweeteners are also offset by a diet which is high in whole foods in general: fresh fruits and vegetables, fresh oils, good quality protein, and, again, whole grains. For, if your diet is weighted in the direction of whole foods, nutritionally speaking, there's definitely room for some refined foods as well. Think of it this way: whole foods are the bookcase and the refined sweets are the knickknacks in the bookcase. The bookcase is the main, supportive structure and the knickknacks are something pretty to liven it up.

When we think about eating sweets, most of us don't think about eating them for nutrition. In fact, we often regard the consumption of sweets as guilty pleasures or as stolen moments during which a type of sleight-of-hand is necessary so that no one sees the piece of candy disappearing into our wide-open mouths. But there's absolutely no reason that we can't have nourishment and pleasure together in the same piece of pie or cake or chocolate. After all, eating for pleasure is extremely important to our short- and long-term health. But most of us tend to eat the type of sweets made with refined sugar and refined flour; and foods high in calories and low in nutrition are something which we can't afford to eat on a regular basis, for we all need the nutrients and most of us don't need the extra calories.

Eating empty calories is hard on us in another, more subtle way: Whole foods have a richness and a nutritional texture to them which our bodies need, not just to survive, but to be vibrant, flexible, and adaptable. A diet high in cardboard calories takes its toll on us in a profound way, for, over time, the body, hungry for the depth of nutrition which it requires, starts to experience a type of low-level starvation. This kind of long-term deprivation makes the body easy fodder for a whole host of medical problems; but it also tends to give the body - as well as the mind, emotions, and spirit - the message that they can never have what they want. A client once said that the idea of eating for nourishment was a revelation to her: in other words, food was her enemy and not her friend. It's easy to feel this way about sweets in particular because we don't usually think of them as foods. And when it comes to sweets made with refined products, this is actually true. They add nothing to our nourishment and are often liabilities. Balancing nutrition and pleasure can be a tricky thing; but there's no reason that sweets can't be our friends. One way to make friends out of them is to think of them in terms of their potential nutritional value and eat sweets made with unrefined and less-refined products. The other way to do this is to, as above, keep refined and processed foods to a minimum and whole foods to a maximum. *

Become your own authority. Finally, and most importantly, do your own research. Give yourself a chance to be aware of the effect that eating sweets has upon you personally. Try to notice how you feel after eating sweets made with different types of refined and less-refined sweeteners. Do you notice a change in your mood or in your staying power? Do you get a sugar high, only to be dropped like a hot potato a few hours later? Do you notice yourself becoming cranky and brittle? Glucose is the fuel of choice for almost all the cells of the body. Refined sugar is very easily and quickly broken down into pure glucose; thus, when we consume a large amount of refined sugar, the effect of having so much available fuel circulating in our bloodstream is to make us feel high. (This sugar high is very similar to the high we experience after drinking coffee, because the caffeine sets off a chain of events which results in the liver dumping pure glucose into the bloodstream.) Then, when our blood sugar level rises above a certain point, the pancreas releases insulin which pulls the sugar molecules out of the bloodstream and we experience a drop in blood sugar - an insulin-induced hypoglycemia which can affect our mood and our sense of physical well-being. In other words, when our blood sugar takes a dip, our mood does as well. This sugar high is something that we usually get only from refined sweeteners; because of its simplicity, the sugar (usually sucrose) molecules are broken down very quickly into glucose and fructose. And because of their uniformity, they're all entering the bloodstream at the same time: Thus, the noticeable spike in our blood sugar followed by the noticeable dip. The biochemical complexity of whole foods allows this to happen more slowly, and allows us to avoid both the sudden rise and the resultant crash.

Try to be aware of what changes, if any, occur in your body or in your mental and emotional states after eating sweets. Each of us is unique and different from every one else - which is what makes this planet such an interesting place on which to live. For some of us, blood sugar is an issue; for others, it's not. Because of our individual energetic and biochemical makeup, some of us have a body chemistry which lends itself to blood-sugar problems, while the body chemistry of others allows them to easily weather the onslaught of donuts, pies, and cakes. And the body we have at any given moment may be vastly different from the body we had yesterday. For our bodies are in a constant state of change. They're continually breaking down old cells and building new ones. They're influenced by the peaks and valleys of hormonal fluctuations, by the sun, the weather and the atmospheric pressure. They're influenced by the quality of the food that we eat, where these foods were grown, and how they were prepared. They're influenced by our mental and emotional state, and the mental and emotional state of those around us. They're influenced by the strength of our spirit - that is, the degree to which we feel connected to others and to everything around us. Applied to the issue of eating sweets, this means that some days we may be able to handle more refined sugar, while a week later eating a Snickers Bar may catapult us into orbit and then leave us feeling jittery, brittle, and crabby.

But I urge you to do some experimentation of your own. There are a lot of unrefined, or less-refined, sweeteners out there, such as maple syrup, barley malt syrup, rice syrup, date sugar, and certain grades of less-refined cane sugar and cane syrup which can be used for sweetening. Some of these, such as honey and maple syrup, are significantly sweeter than refined sugar, while some of them, such as brown rice syrup and barley malt syrup, are significantly less sweet. Fruit juices also make wonderful sweeteners. They contain a tremendous amount of naturally-occurring sugar (mostly sucrose, or glucose joined to fructose), which seems obvious if you think of how many apples it takes to make one glass of juice. (The next time you down a nice big glass of orange juice, you might want to think about this. Your liver might thank you.) However, 'modified' fruit juice concentrates have usually been processed in a way which removes most of their nutrients and makes them more like refined sugar and less like a whole food. Adding whole fruit to cakes and quick breads allows you to decrease the amount of sweetener while increasing their nutritional value. There's also a sweetener called agave nectar, which is made from the Blue Agave plant, a relative of aloe vera. Agave nectar is about thirty percent sweeter than granulated sugar, but I think the main inducement to trying it is that is just sounds so sensual and exotic.

Personally, my two favorites are grade B maple syrup and agave nectar. Even though grade A is obviously considered to be a superior product, I prefer grade B. It hasn't undergone as much processing as grade A and so it has more of a mapley taste; and I love the gentle way it sweetens coffee and chocolate and the fact that it doesn't leave a residue or aftertaste in your mouth the way refined sugar does. In the sugar wars, it's been said that there's no difference in the rate at which unrefined and refined sweeteners break down in the body. But my experience of my own personal body says that this is not true, that there *is* a significant difference in the way I feel after eating refined sugar and the way I feel after eating maple syrup.

Agave nectar tastes to me like a spicy honey and it doesn't seem to give that sugar rush of other sweeteners - something that is most noticeable with refined sugar, where its effect can be like that of a drug. At least to me. I use it in coffee and to sweeten up brown rice after it's been cooked. It's pretty good in oatmeal, but I still prefer tree sap (maple syrup).

(A word of caution here: Please do not give honey to a child two years old or younger. In its natural state, honey has a certain amount of bacteria; the immature immune systems of infants and small children are not capable of handling this, and so the results can be quite severe. Most of the honey on the market has been heated in order to kill bacteria, but the dangers of ingesting unheated honey - because of a labeling error, for instance - are too great to take a chance. Check with your pediatrician if you need further information.)

There are also synthetic sweeteners, such as aspartame, which is created by joining together two amino acids (the building blocks of proteins). The attraction of something like aspartame is that it has no calories; but, to my mind, the idea of a synthetic sweetener is much nicer than the reality. For, once again, the Caveperson Factor applies, and giving our caveperson-era bodies something which was created only a few decades ago is probably asking for trouble. It's often challenging to be a human being in the twenty-first century, where technology zooms past our very ancient physical reality. But, once again, the basis of health is to cultivate a compassionate approach to ourselves. And so, faced with something like aspartame which seems to answer the desire many of us have - to have our cake and to eat it too - it's good to try to accept the fact that the home of our twenty-first-century minds is something which is actually very old. Using a 'modern' sweetener like aspartame on a regular basis is most likely asking for trouble because the body probably hasn't a clue what to do with it.

But I urge you to draw your own conclusions. Do your own research. Go to your local natural foods store or to the natural foods section in your supermarket and see what they have. One of the attractions of refined sugar is that it doesn't have a strong, characteristic taste the way maple syrup does, and so you may need to try a few sweeteners before you find one that you like. When dealing with matters of health, it's easy to fall into the trap of confusing good health with "being good". "Being good" usually means embracing a set of rules and berating or punishing ourselves when we fail to follow them. During this time of sweetness, allow the harmony and strength of the season to support you. Let it help steer you away from the precarious peaks of 'good' and 'bad' and toward the openheartedness of being good to yourself. Trusting yourself to make your own decisions and be your own authority is something which increases your level of health and well-being. It's also something which increases your level of internal security, for it means that you trust yourself to be your own mother, that loving and caring presence who is always there for you, taking care of you and doing things which are good for you. It *is* possible to have taste and nutrition. It *is* possible to have sweetness which adds something to your life. So during this season when the Siren of Sweetness calls to you, let yourself answer.

🪷 Digestion

The season of late summer is an expression of the energy of the earth element. In acupuncture school, we were taught that the best way to learn about the elements is to go out into nature and observe them. So, let's go outside and look at the earth. What do we see? Well, first of all, we see something horizontal, something flat, something that is lying there, passive and inert. We see something that is physically supporting us, holding us up. We see something that is physically supporting and nourishing green, growing things. A twig falls onto the earth. Let's watch for a few minutes to see what happens. . . . Well, actually, *nothing* is happening. The earth has accepted the twig and given it a resting-place. The twig hasn't been thrown back at the tree or moved to another spot on the ground. And, looking at the other objects which have fallen onto the ground, we can see what will happen to the twig after it has lain there for days or weeks or months. We can see that the twig, like the tree branches, the flower petals, acorns, cigarette butts and candy wrappers, will rot and break down into smaller and smaller pieces until it is finally transformed into soil. We can see that there's a process which somehow changes that which we know as "twig" into something completely different - and thus unrecognizable - from its original, twiggy nature: soil, earth, the ground beneath our feet, our foundation, our mother, our home and our final resting place. And we can see that all the other objects will undergo the same process. The branches, the candy wrappers, the seeds, the acorns, the cigarette remains, even the bottle caps will finally be dissolved and changed into the cool, firm bosom of mother Earth.

Digestion is a process of transformation. It's the series of steps which allows us to take something separate from us

- something which is *not* us - and make it into something which is part of us - something which *is* us. It's the process by which we take bigger things and break them down into smaller things in order to get to the nutrients inside, and so it's the process by which we nourish ourselves. On the physical level, then, digestion allows us to take something growing in a field and make it into a skin or kidney cell. On the mental level, digestion allows us to watch the news and come up with a theory about political or socioeconomic trends. On the emotional level, digestion allows us to listen to another human being - or to ourselves - and to understand why they're so upset and angry. On a more global level, digestion is a process which links us to our environment, our planet, and our world.

Chinese and western medicine converge at certain points, but in general they're vastly different from each other. In Chinese medicine, the stomach and the spleen are the two officials responsible for digestion, whereas in western medicine, the organs of digestion are the stomach, the small intestine, the large intestine, the pancreas, the liver, and the gall bladder. (The mouth, the salivary glands, the esophagus, and the pharynx are the other components of the digestive tract.) Because it's based upon the physical reality, western medicine focusses a great deal of attention on the anatomy of an organ - that is, what the organ looks like and how it's constructed on the macroscopic and microscopic levels. But Chinese medicine is based upon the concept of energy; and, according to this concept, an organ is simply one of the physical expressions of a certain type of energy. Thus, in Chinese medicine an organ's anatomy is unimportant (and actually never discussed), but there's a great deal of discussion focussed on its function, or physiology. Let's use an example from another season and another element: the gallbladder. In western medicine, the gall bladder is a small, green, pear-shaped sac attached to the surface of the liver and its functions are to store, concentrate, and release bile into the small intestine. But in Chinese medicine, the gall bladder is considered to be one of the twelve officials, and an official is much, much more than an organ. (Ancient China was governed by a vast and complex bureaucracy; hence the term "official".) Each of the officials is actually an elemental correspondence, an expression of a specific elemental energy. The ancient Chinese who synthesized the system known as the Five Elements saw the officials as a family of twelve little people inside of us, each with his or her own unique personality and each with duties and responsibilities that only he or she could carry out. Once again, both the personality and the duties of a particular official are expressions of a particular elemental energy. Thus, the quick-witted, enthusiastic, "can-do!" gallbladder official is one of the voices of the creative, goal-oriented energy of the wood element. The gallbladder is a peppy little thing; it's ability to be focussed and its facility for quick response and split-second-timing allow it to do what none of the other eleven officials can: function as the designated decision-maker of the body, mind, spirit, and emotions. For the gallbladder is responsible for getting us down the path of life from point A to point B. As partner to the liver (the designated planner of the energy system), the gallbladder's job is to execute the liver's plans and make them into realities.

And so the stomach official is much more than simply the large, muscular sac at the end of the esophagus. It's the part of us which takes everything in and equalizes it. Just like the earth which accepts everything and turns nothing

54

away, the stomach works democratically to take things which are quite different from each other and to make them all the same. Facts, sights, sounds, smells, food, drink, medications, the emotions and opinions of others, diesel fumes and the sky at sunset - everything goes into the great mixing bowl that is the stomach and gets processed along with everything else. The stomach is also the great integrator and unifier. For in order to make it through one single, ordinary day here on planet Earth, we have to deal with a world of facts, objects, beliefs, sensations, emotions, and ideas; and the stomach is the part of the energy system which allows us to bring together these unrelated - and often warring - elements and mix them up into a single, unified whole. The energy of the earth element is the energy of the mother; and the stomach is very much like a mother who stands with arms open wide, ready to include whatever and whomever steps into the welcoming circle of her embrace. And it's this accepting, nonjudgmental energy which allows us to combine the argument we had with our husband, the chocolate cake we had for breakfast, and the 7:00 a.m. news into something that seems reasonable and acceptable. Thus, the stomach official is the part of the energy system which allows us to interact with the world around us without feeling constantly overwhelmed and on the verge of a nervous breakdown. But the stomach is not only the great integrator and equalizer, it's also the great dismantler. For the stomach allows us to take the food, the drink, the medications, the sensations, the fumes, the sunset, and the information and, through a process of rotting and ripening, break it all down into smaller, more digestible bits. The stomach's power to dismantle - like its powers to equalize and unify - is something which allows us to make sense of our existence and our world. For example, the energy of the stomach official is what allows us to take the the hour or two of murder and assorted mayhem, politics, recipes, weather reports, movie reviews, interviews, and fashion trends - in other words, the 7 a.m. news - and break it all down into its components parts in order to make sense of it and understand it.

Thus the stomach official is the great mixing bowl. It's the receptacle which holds the batter which the stomach itself has created through its powers of integration, equalization, and dismantling. And when the batter is just right, when it's been ripened and broken down enough, the stomach hands the batter over to that great transformer - the spleen - and the spleen changes it into something completely different from its original nature. Thus, if the stomach official is the part of the energy system which takes disparate ingredients and mixes them up into a nice, uniform batter, then the spleen official is the part of the energy system which transforms the mixture of flour, milk, eggs, honey, and vanilla into the birthday treat that we call "cake". Through its powers of transformation, the spleen takes what the stomach has processed and changes it into something else, something different from its original nature, something which will nourish our bodies, our minds, our spirits, and our emotions. The spleen is the part of the energy system which allows us to make liver cells out of spaghetti and the theory of relativity out of mathematical equations. It's the part of the energy system which allows us to take those dismantled bits and pieces of the morning news and make them into something else: an idea or opinion, for example, a song or a poem. Thus, the stomach is our link to the present, while the spleen is our link to what lies ahead.

Late summer is the transition time of the year. It's the bridge between the boisterous activity of the first part of the year (spring and summer) and the peace and quiet of the second (fall and winter); and the ability to digest our lives is one of the things which makes this transition possible. For the energy of late summer asks us to sit and muse and mull things over; its great golden embrace offers us the time and the place to take apart the preceding months and years, to break it down into smaller, more understandable bits, and to transform it into something that will sustain us. Who we are at any moment is the culmination of everything we have experienced, felt, thought or done in our lives, and so who we are changes from moment to moment. The digestive nature of late summer allows us to transform all that we now find ourselves to be into something which will support and nourish us in the coming months and years. Just like the earth which takes twig and leaf, candywrapper and cigarette butt and converts all of it into something which grows oak trees and berry bushes, our own stomach and spleen energy allows us to take the events, thoughts, deeds, emotions, and sensations of the past months and years and change it into something which will feed us. For example, you may have lost a loved one in the past months or years, and you may never have given yourself the chance to digest this, to take it apart and break it down into its component parts. Losing someone who is close to you can be devastating, and the thought of sitting down in order to process this may be far from appealing. In fact, it may seem terrifying and too overwhelming to even consider. Yet losing a loved one is a lot to digest. It's a change which is felt in every aspect of one's life and at a very profound level. Giving yourself over to the task of processing all of this may seem daunting, but the reality is that *not* making the time and space for doing this is usually much more injurious to one's physical, mental, emotional, and spirit-level health. And you might find, after taking it all apart and looking at it, that there's something in the experience which will nourish you. You might find that, like the first flowers of spring poking up through the snow, the experience has given you a greater sense of spiritual awareness. Or you may find that, surprise of surprises, you feel less fearful about life and death rather than the opposite.

So during this season of nourishment and transformation, give yourself the gift of digestion. This is the transition time of the year, and so it can be a time when we feel unsettled and our lives feel disjointed to us. Because the energy of late summer is one which includes everything and leaves nothing out, this can also be a time of year when we can feel pulled in many directions and lose our ability to feel centered and grounded. Take a moment here or there - or an entire afternoon or day or week, if you want to and you can - and give yourself time to process your life. The world is changing at a pace which can sometimes feel overwhelming, and we're all changing with it. Let yourself have the opportunity to make some sense of all of this. Start by allowing yourself to be aware of what's going on around you at this very moment. This will help center you and allow you to see who you are, and what your life is, at this moment in time. The energy of late summer is the energy of the physical, so the act of noticing - the act of really trying to see - the physical world helps get us here into the present. As human beings, we tend to feel that the physical reality is the most important reality; but we also tend to sail through the physical and interact with it without really seeing it in a certain way. Looking at a chair, for example, and trying to take in its presence through the eyes; trying to see how it's 'giving' its weight to the floor, how it's resting on the floor and how the floor is holding up the chair - this is very different from using your sight to ascertain whether there's a chair in the room and where, exactly, it is. Using our eyes to take in the reality which is there in front of us instead of using them to confirm the reality which we expect to see helps ground us in the present and allows us to be present. So, if you're outside, try to notice what's going on in your back yard or on the street in front of your house. What are the trees doing? Is the light shining through their leaves? What does the sun feel like? Is there a breeze? How does it feel against your skin? Are there birds? What are they doing? What are the plants doing? How do they look? Notice how the buildings are sitting on the ground. Notice how the ground is holding up the buildings. If you're inside, try to notice how the chair you're sitting in feels against your body or how solid the floor feels beneath your feet. What is the light like? What color are the walls of the room you're sitting in? Color changes with the light, so even though you know that they were painted a certain color, what color are the walls right now?

And now try to notice what's going on in the world inside of you. Just try to focus inward and be with all of it for a second or two. It's easy to get distracted, but that's just a natural part of having a brain. If your mind gets pulled to those bills that need paying or the calls you have to make, allow yourself to focus again on the teeming, swirling, colorful world inside of you. Try to be with all of its activity, its sound and its motion, for a few more moments. Then try to let yourself be with everything that's going on inside of you and everything that's going on around you in its totality. Just for a second or two, try to suspend judgment. Yes, it's not the happiest thing in the world that the paint is peeling off the front door or that there's a new spider condo in the living room. But just try to be with all of this all at once and see how it feels. There's something very comforting and sweet in allowing yourself the time and the space to sit with the whole mix of events and sensations that is your life. And there's something grounding in giving yourself a break from taking in new input so that you can process what you've already taken in. You may notice how much movement there is within the stillness you've created. Or something, a thought or an emotion, may bubble to the surface of your consciousness. It may be something that you haven't totally digested yet. Perhaps it's something from your past; perhaps someone had hurt you, or you them. Or perhaps you've been working on forgiving someone for something, but you haven't been able to get to a point of completion yet - and perhaps you never will. Perhaps you've been working toward some kind of success and you're afraid you'll never get there. Or perhaps you've had a wonderful year so far, or a wonderful last few years, and what's coming up is a sense of happiness. None of this matters. The energy of late summer is not one that helps us complete or finish things; it's not an energy which helps us define things as good or bad, happy or sad so we can then know which way to go. It's not an energy for making decisions or for establishing the worth of things. It's not an energy that allows us to establish relationships or make them better. It's an energy that supports breaking things down. It's an energy that allows us to take things apart in order to get to the nutrients inside. It's an energy which allows us to transform pieces of our environment into pieces of ourselves. It's an energy which allows us to transform the pieces of our lives into something sweet and nourishing. It's an energy which asks us to acknowledge who we are at this very moment, and so it's an energy which allows us to ground and center ourselves. So let the thoughts come, let the emotions come, let the paint peel and the spider spin its web. There will always be happiness in life, there will always be sadness. There will be misery and failure, triumph and fulfillment. It's all part of this great, spiraling, wild and crazy ride that we call life, and late summer gives us the groundedness - and the taste buds - to let it nourish us. ✔ ✔

❦ Care and Feeding of the Sinuses

From the viewpoint of western medicine, the sinuses are hollow cavities in the bones of the skull. They form a ring around the nasal cavities and produce mucus which drains into them. The sinuses act to give our voices more resonance and lighten the skull; but, beyond that, they seem to serve no other function. But in Chinese medicine, the sinuses are much more than that. In Chinese medicine, the sinuses are an integral part of the process of digestion. For the sinuses assist in our ability to digest things on the nonphysical level and are part of the mechanism by which we take in information. And this information can be in the form of words and facts which we hear or read; it can be auditory stimuli such as noise, music and other sounds, or visual stimulation such as movies, books, magazines, or TV; it can be environmental input such as construction and traffic noise; or it can be information on other levels, such as the emotional energy and thoughts of others. Problems with the sinuses, such as congestion and headache, are often the result of taking in too much information and not having the time, or the space, in which to process it. Sometimes, when we're already depleted or when we've been bombarded with too much input for too long a time, the sinus overload can become so severe that the symptoms mimic those of a sinus infection. And sometimes chronically overloaded sinuses can be a contributing factor to a real, *bona fide* sinus infection which requires antibiotics to cure it.

Seasons are times of year when the energy of a certain element pulsates most strongly. And when the pulsation of a certain type of energy is at its peak, the energy pulsating through all of its expressions is strongest as well, illuminating them and making them stand out. This means that, during late summer, all the expressions of the earth element have the loudest voice, and you may notice an increase in sinus sensitivity, congestion, and pain. But it also means that it's the time of year when it will be easiest to understand what's causing these symptoms and how to make yourself feel better. Here are a few ideas to get you started:

(1) **Drink enough water.** Energetically speaking, the sinuses are involved in digestion, (See the "Water It " heading in the "Body" section.) and being properly hydrated is indispensable to the digestive process. So, if you find yourself the lucky recipient of a sinus headache, try drinking a glass or two or three of water and see if that helps.

(2) **Check your diet.** Often, the same foods which we have trouble digesting are also the cause of nasal and sinus congestion. Dairy products such as milk and cheese can also be the cause of nasal and sinus congestion, although yogurt, another dairy product, seems to be a special case. Some of us who have trouble with dairy don't have the same difficulty with yogurt. This may be due to the fact that yogurt contains live bacterial cultures which act to repopulate the digestive tract and actually aid in the digestive process.

(3) **Check caffeine usage**. Caffeine makes us feel omnipotent. It makes us feel as though we can do anything and that we have no limitations. But caffeine also makes it possible for us to override the body's signals which tell us to stop, sit down, and take a break. And when we're not getting the message from ourselves

that says, "I can't take anymore", we push ourselves past the limit and end up putting ourselves in situations where we have to take in even more.

(4) Check your intake of refined sugar. Eating a lot (whatever that means for you) of refined sugar and drinking caffeine have the same end result: a great deal of pure glucose enters the bloodstream all at once, raising our blood sugar level quickly and giving us that sugar high.

(5) Try to avoid blowing your nose. The mucus produced in the nasal cavities traps foreign invaders such as bacteria. Blowing your nose creates a type of back pressure which can actually force some of these things - things which most of us would rather not think about - back up into the nasal passages; and because the sinuses drain into the nasal passages, this can interfere with sinus drainage. Blowing your nose also irritates the tissue that lines the nasal passages; and since the mucosa which line the nasal passages and the sinuses is continuous, what happens in the nasal passages has an effect upon the sinuses as well. (The mucosa lining the sinuses is actually continuous throughout the entire respiratory tract, including the sinuses, the nasal passages, and the tear ducts.) Just let your nose run and dab gently with a tissue or handkerchief. Blowing usually creates a vicious circle: Blowing creates more irritation. More irritation creates more mucus. More mucus leads to more blowing. So less blowing almost always lessens the *need* to blow.

(6) Finally, let the symptom be your friend. If you find yourself becoming congested or getting a sinus headache, take a moment. Stop. Pull back from what you're doing and ask yourself how you're feeling. Often when the stomach official is on overload, it feels as though we just can't take anymore. There's an acupuncture point on the stomach meridian called "Abundant Splendor", and, in a very specific way, "Abundant Splendor" is a perfect description of the season of late summer. For this is the time of year when the Earth showers us with her incredible abundance, when she gives to us everything we need and plenty of it. Because the stomach is in charge of taking in all of this bounty, it's just as possible to feel overwhelmed by the happy as by the sad. The point "Abundant Splendor" awakens the ability within our energy systems to digest everything that we've taken in. So, during this season of abundance, listen to what your sinuses are telling you and, if you can, give yourself a moment of "Abundant Splendor". Take a few minutes or a couple of hours, a day or a week and allow yourself the time that you need to break everything down and make it part of you. ✒ ✒

✹ Till the Soil

Each season has something specific to teach us, a lesson, if you will, a gift from that season's core. The downward movement of fall teaches us how to let go, while winter's watery darkness shows us how to have faith; the anger which we feel in springtime teaches us how to forgive, while summer's warmth and light shows us that we must give up the need for control in order to merge with others; and late summer, that time of needs in the midst of abundance and generosity, teaches us how to be of service. The soil is a perfect expression of this, for the soil serves. And soil is an amazing thing, a mind-bogglingly intricate substance formed by the intersection of many different energies: the chemical and mechanical effects of sun, wind, humidity; the flow of water and air; the interplay of ions such as iron, magnesium, and aluminum; the teeming activity of microorganisms which break down and transform plant and animal remains; the burrowing of small mammals, earthworms, and insects; and the passage of time.

So during this season of service, give yourself the opportunity to be of service to something which serves us all the time. Do some weeding. Pick a piece of garden or yard that's two feet by two feet and weed it. Even if it's not your job, or even if you never intend to do it again, give yourself a chance to give to the earth (and to the Earth) in the way that it gives to us. Pick up a trowel or other weeding implement. Dig in the soil. Use your hands if you want to. Pull out the bermuda grass and the unwanted volunteers. Give yourself a chance to do what the tunnelers and the borers do -- aerate and cultivate the soil, move it around, mix together the mineral and the organic components, and improve its health and its fertility. The earth is a humble substance; it's something that we walk upon all the time. Give yourself the opportunity to have an experience of your own humility in a way that feeds you, in a way that allows you to connect with your own energy of late summer. I'm not trying to romanticize weeding. I don't shout for joy and cry "Yippeeeee!!!" when I look out at my garden and see the fish pond disappearing under chickweed and dandelions. Weeding is work, and often it's hard work. But if you've never given yourself a chance to experience the soil in this way, now's the time. Go on out there, out into the gentle strength of late summer. Add your energy to that of the the burrowers, the tillers, and the movers -- the moles and the voles, the ants, and the earthworms. Add your movement to that of the water and the air, the ions, the sun, and the passage of time. Hang out with the bacteria and the fungi. (Wear a dust mask if you need to.) See what the experience has to offer you; and, even if it's not your cup of tea, allow it to nourish and strengthen you by teaching you how to serve. ✕ ✕

🌺 Do Something Nice For Your Feet

In many ways, the feet are an expression of the energy of the earth element, for just like the earth beneath us, we walk on them, and they support us. And the human foot is a unique and wondrous thing; for our desire as a race to stand and walk upright - and, unlike other mammals, to do it all the time - subjects our feet to a tremendous amount of stress. Because impact is a combination of body weight and intensity of force, a 120-pound person subjects each foot to 180 pounds of force with walking, and 300 to 360 pounds with running. It's estimated that, over the course of a lifetime, the 'average' person walks about 75,000 to 150,000 miles (300,000 for a professional athlete) and, according to the U. S. Department of Labor, every day takes 18,000 steps, thereby moving two to three million pounds of his or her own weight on a daily basis.

Those of us who are able to walk ask a lot of our feet, but the feet are up to the challenge, for the feet are complex, sturdy, and accommodating. Each foot has twenty-eight bones, fifty-six ligaments, thirty-eight muscles, and thirty-five joints which are lined with cartilage and lubricated with synovial fluid. This collection of bones, muscles, ligaments, and joints - and the attendant blood vessels and nerves - is organized in several different ways to allow the foot to accomplish all that it has to do. For, within the skin of each unassuming foot, many different lines of energy are running, forming several different patterns which swirl through it simultaneously.

First, there are three different regions of the foot - the hindfoot, midfoot, and forefoot - which perform different tasks, from shock absorption and stabilization to propulsion and flexibility. Next, the 28 bones and 112 ligaments form four arches, and these also have different functions which range from support to shock absorption to adjusting to uneven surfaces. And then there are the toes. The big toe is large and solid, with only two phalanges or toe bones, while the other four are much smaller and have three phalanges apiece. The differences in anatomy between the big toe and the other four is due to the fact that they also have different jobs: the big toe is built for shouldering the majority of the body's weight, while the function of the other four is primarily to add spring to our step. Part of the foot's complexity is due to the fact that half of its bones do double duty, and are therefore part of more than one of these patterns. Thus, for instance, the metatarsals are part of the forefoot and, as such, are responsible for propulsion. But they are also part of the anterior metatarsal arch which allows the foot to adjust to uneven surfaces. (One of the more fascinating things about the big toe is that, embedded in the tendons at its base[1] are two tiny sesamoid bones. In the human body, sesamoid bones are unique because they are not connected to the rest of the skeleton in the way that other bones are; but these tiny little bones, which are the approximate shape and size of sesame seeds, are vital to our ability to move around, for, together with other bones and their attendant soft tissues, they form a type of block and tackle system which allows us to raise and lower our big toe, among other things.)

Energy is constantly flowing into us from the planet. If you'd like to see where this is happening, sit down, pick up one of your feet, and turn it over so that you're looking at the sole. Flex your toes toward you (use your hand to do this if you need to) and look for the depression on the ball

---

1 i.e., in the head of the first metatarsal

of your foot that's in line with the space between your second and third toes. This point, called "Bubbling Spring", is part of an energy center which allows us to connect with the energy of the planet. But energy is also flowing out of us and back into the Earth. In the foot, as in the rest of the body, energy follows the contours of our anatomy. Like water flowing along a river bed, our energy follows the natural channels formed by bones, joints, ligaments, tendons, and muscles. Thus, when the anatomy of the foot is temporarily changed by wearing shoes that squeeze our toes together or 4-inch spike heels which change the weight distribution in the foot and put pressure on parts that can't really handle it, we change the flow of energy through the foot as well. The movement of energy within the foot is compromised, and the movement of energy into the foot and out of the foot is compromised as well. Even worse, prolonged foot abuse can change the anatomy of the foot permanently; and, when this happens, the flow of energy through the foot is altered or compromised in a way which is also permanent. And because our energy systems, like our bodies, are ecologies, a change in the flow of energy through the foot means a change in the flow of energy through the entire body. Bunions, for example, are deformities caused in part by wearing shoes that are too tight around the toes. (People who develop bunions are also structurally predisposed to them, so shoe fit is just one of the factors in acquiring them.) Another permanent change in the foot's anatomy is "fallen arches", a flattening of the foot due to a weakening of the ligaments which hold the heel and the front of the foot together. Those of us who have to be on our feet for prolonged periods of time are more susceptible to this problem. Because each twenty pounds of body weight becomes thirty pounds with each step that we take, those of us who gain too much weight can suffer from persistent foot pain which, over time, can successfully kill the joy of walking, or of being on our feet at all. Very often, human females have a special relationship to their feet which often seems to predispose them to foot abuse. Because small, dainty feet are still associated with femininity, many of us are, even now in the twenty-first century, squishing our feet into shoes which restrict the flow of energy through the foot. The story of Cinderella says it all. The original tale, as told by the Brothers Grimm, is really a story about virtue and its rewards in which the female foot has a pivotal role. Cinderella, who was good, had small feet, while her stepsisters, who were evil, had feet which were much larger. Both stepsisters were successful in getting their feet into the slipper but had to cut off a piece of foot in order to do it; luckily (?) the blood flowing out of the slipper gave them away. Cinderella's goodness was rewarded with happiness and status, while her two evil stepsisters, as their reward, were blinded by birds.

The foot is an expression of the energy of support; and so when we affect our feet in ways that cause pain, discomfort, or damage, we're directly affecting our own energy of support and our ability to be supportive of ourselves. So, during this time of year when the energy of support is at its peak, you can increase your own energy of support by giving some attention to your feet. Here are some suggestions:

Exercise them to stretch and strengthen the muscles in the foot and ankle. Because the foot is so complex, one would expect exercises for them to be complex as well, but they're not. Here are a few:

(1) Sit down and, with your bare feet, try to pick up a bath towel or a pencil.

(2) Stand on the floor and raise up and down on your toes five to ten times.

(3) Sitting on a a soft surface, touch the soles of your feet together.

(4) Take off your shoes and pump your feet. (Pretend to be pumping the gas pedal of your car.) This helps to fluff up the circulation in your calves and feet, and so it feels especially wonderful after you've been standing on them for a long time.

(5) Do this three times: Sit with your legs extended in front of you. Breathe in and, as you do so, flex your feet back toward you as far as you can comfortably - that is, without straining. Then breathe out and point them away from you. (Think of your breath moving your feet if this helps.) Because the flow of energy follows the anatomy, it's greatly affected by that anatomy. Thus, when we stand or walk in ways which alter our energy's normal flow, the flow of energy through the foot and leg can become stuck. We also store energy in our bodies, the energy of thoughts or emotions that we don't know what to do with; and for many of us, that place is the leg, ankle, or foot. So, when you're doing this exercise, as you point your toes, think of breathing the energy all the way down your thigh and your calf, through your foot, and out the toes. It's entirely possible to use your awareness and your breath to move your own energy. Energy travels in spirals; so, if it's helpful to you, think of the energy as a spiral the size and shape of your leg and see the energy spiraling down through the leg and out through the foot. If this doesn't work for you, do what ballet dancers do: Point your toes by pointing your entire leg. In other words, think of the action of pointing your toes as something which originates high up in the leg and not in the toes themselves.

(6) Walk. Because the feet are an expression of the energy of the earth element, the action of walking - that is, giving your entire weight to each foot as it makes contact with the bosom of mother Earth - is an excellent way to both exercise your feet and tone up your earth element energy while doing it. So try to include some walking into your daily or weekly life. Even if you're someone whose exercise regimen includes more strenuous sports, such as running, competitive cycling or swimming, walking is important to the long-term health of your feet. And runners have a special need to walk; for running subjects each foot to an incredible amount of stress and walking is the best way to strengthen them. ✗

Give yourself a foot bath. Soaking your feet in warm water can be very soothing and relaxing, especially when your feet are tired or aching. Adding Epsom salts (a compound which reduces inflammation) or herbs to the water can help even more. Herbs which soothe are lavender, chamomile, rose petals, lemon balm, and lemon verbena. Herbs which revitalize and energize are peppermint and rosemary. Oats or oat straw are wonderful if your feet are itchy because of dry skin. Try a handful of any of these in a basin or a bathtub of water. I personally recommend the lavender, chamomile, and rose petal foot bath. (You may want to put the herbs in a cloth bag before putting them in the water.) ✑

Get a foot massage - or give yourself one. Late summer is the time of both sensuality and caretaking, so it's the perfect time to give your feet, and your self, extra attention. Here are some tips in case you need them: Turn your foot over and rest it on your knee. Take your thumbs and, pressing gently but firmly, walk them over the parts of the foot which bear most of the weight. For most of us, the weight-bearing parts of the foot are the parts which leave a footprint, and the non-weight-bearing parts are the parts which do not. Start with the ball of the foot. Try to press in between the bones there, the five metatarsals which connect to the five toes. (Massaging in places such as these not only helps to increase circulation, it also helps to release energy which may be trapped or sluggish.) Don't neglect the metatarsal heads, the bumpy part of the ball of the foot at the base of the toes. Next, grasp your heel in your hand and squeeze. With your thumb and forefinger, squeeze the outer part of the sole of your foot (the part which is in line with your two smallest toes) from the base all the way up along its length. Now focus on the non-weight-bearing parts. Take your thumbs and, again pressing firmly but gently, run them together up the center of the sole of the foot from the heel to the ball. Using one thumb, press and massage the spot in the middle of the sole which is in line with the leg. This 'bliss spot' (you'll understand if you find it) is part of the transverse arch, the portion of the foot which accepts the weight of the body as it comes down the leg. Then, with your thumb and forefinger, grasp the Achilles tendon, the thick cord which runs along the back of the heel and attaches the heel to muscles in the calf; try to grasp as much of the Achilles tendon as you can and squeeze gently but firmly upward, along its length. Finally, squeeze each toe from the base to the tip, and then put your feet up, lean back, and give yourself a few moments.

We sometimes feel the need to justify giving to ourselves by saying that we've earned it, we're worth it, or we deserve it. But what about the times in our lives when we just need something? Do we need justification in order to give ourselves what we need? Each of us has within us the energies of all five elements. Thus, within each of us is the energy of the kind and giving mother. Often we feel uncomfortable giving to ourselves because we don't have the best relationship with the mother inside; but taking a few minutes to do something nice for your feet is one way of strengthening this inner bond. Giving to the self can be difficult when we've built an entire lifetime around the idea of withholding from the self instead of giving to it; but, during this time of year when mother Earth is giving to *us* so generously, I ask you to take this small, yet significant step toward doing just that. ♪♪

The earth is the place to which we always turn,
the mother who always waits for us,
the cool hand on the fevered brow, the soft voice in
the terrified night,
that which, within and without, is always there
to hold us, to feed us, to comfort us,
and to rock us,
gently, gently, gently back to sleep,
the hand whose soft touch launches us into the
moonlit shining boat of dreamland,
the sweet dense home to which everything -
all that was given and all that was given back,
all the love, all the hatred,
all the words spoken in kindness and all those that cut
like glass,
the truths, the lies, the dreams, the despair,
the first baby teeth and the bones returning to dust -
all come home, all have a place, all come to rest,
equal and equalized within her cool, dark, and
moldering breast.

☸ Insecurity

The Earth is one of the supreme expressions of the energy of the earth element and thus of the energy of late summer. Because it's a sphere that spins on its axis and orbits the sun, life on planet Earth is something that often repeats itself: days become nights and then days again, winter winds its way into summer and then, before you know it, it's time to haul out the heavy coats one more time. This quality of repeating something over and over again can be a source of mind-numbing monotony, but it can also act as a salve to soothe the terrors and frustrations of life on planet Earth. Take the issue of time, for example. The concept of time, and whether it is real or simply an illusion, is something which has been discussed and argued about for centuries by scientists, philosophers, and spiritual teachers. But when we're down in the trenches of life, all of us - and I mean all of us - feel the press time. We all feel it pulling us forward, dragging us away from a past that is known and familiar, and toward a future that is unknown, mysterious, and often frightening. And this is something which can make us feel nervous and insecure. But the cycles of life tell us that day comes after night and spring follows winter. The cycles of life tell us, "Even though it's dark now, it will be light again. Even though it's cold now, the sun will return to warm us." The cycles of life, the reality of something which returns and which brings us back to a certain point over and over again, is something that can calm our fears, settle our nerves, and give us a way to center ourselves. The cyclical nature of life on Earth tells us that there is always another tomorrow and always another chance.

Late summer is the time of year when the cyclical nature of life is most strongly felt. The cycles of the Earth, as well as the biological cycles of all plant and animal life on the Earth, are expressions of the energy of the earth element. And because late summer is the time when the energy of the earth element reigns supreme, it's the time of year when the energies of security and its evil twin, insecurity, are most profoundly felt. Thus, during late summer, you may find yourself feeling overly worried about your personal safety. You may find yourself checking the doors on your house or office several times to make sure that they are actually, definitely, and definitively locked. You may find yourself feeling overly concerned about what others think about you; you may catch yourself spending a great deal of time, for instance, wondering whether the boy who just bagged your groceries thinks that you're a nice person. Or you may notice that this is a time of year when your need to be mothered is at its peak and that you really, really, really need someone to take care of you, fix you a nice dinner, and tuck you in at night - literally and/or figuratively.

What is insecurity, then? It's a type of internal homelessness, a feeling of not belonging, a feeling of not being connected to the central point of who we are. When we move, for example, we experience this type of disconnection - which is precisely why moving is such such a living hell. For when we're moving, we're in between residences; and so, for the time being at least, home - that place where we go to get our bearings, that place where we go to collapse and replenish ourselves, the place that is always there for us, the place that says "This is where you belong" - does not exist. The energy which we know as 'home' is the energy of a contained, warm coziness, and feeling secure means feeling at home within ourselves; it means feeling supported at our core. Often, many of us are very good at creating this type of support on an external level; we have friends, family, and even a work life that nourishes and sustains us. But this only goes so far. At some point, we need to learn to do this for ourselves, because the ability to give our*selves* support for who we are is indispensable to developing a sense of internal security. Constantly looking outside ourselves for anything is something that pulls us away from our core and throws us off balance. Constantly focussing beyond ourselves for those things we feel we don't have - approval, validation, The Answer - eventually leaves us feeling insecure in the same way that little children do when their mothers aren't around. Tiny little children need to look outside themselves for help and support because they are literally unable to take care of themselves. And so when mother is away or even in the next room, they can experience fear and a deep sense of insecurity because their central point of reference, their giver of food and life and warmth, is gone. And we all have this part within us. In our culture, describing someone as insecure is usually meant as a criticism. This is because the insecurity of others reminds us only too well of our own insecurity, and our own insecurity is something which terrifies us. Like the frightened three-year-old who needs mama to take care of him or her, we often feel unable to fend for ourselves against the cruelties and vagaries of life. And, like the frightened three-year-old, we often have not developed a way of giving ourselves the kind of internal support which makes us feel that we're standing on a firm foundation instead of a shaky one.

In the cycle of the seasons, late summer is the time of year when the energies of support and security, and their counterparts, lack of support and insecurity, are strongest; thus it's the time of year when it's easiest to see and understand our own insecurities and how to heal them. Take some time during this season and ask yourself what makes you feel insecure? Do you feel unsure of your ability to push your life forward in the direction that you want it to go? Do you feel unsure of your words or your actions and find yourself adjusting your behavior and what you say in order to please others and/or gain their approval and support? Perhaps you're someone who has been able to create a life for yourself in which you feel in charge of things and secure, yet the idea of not knowing how to do something -set up a new computer system, for instance - makes you feel as though there's an earthquake inside of you, ready to shake you into so many pieces. There's no shame in having insecurities. Inside all of us, there's a three-year-old who would like nothing more than to hide behind mother's skirt and hold on to her leg for dear life. And what do three-year-olds need when they're feeling frightened and insecure? Comfort and support. Yet what we usually give these parts of ourselves is not comfort and support but criticism, harsh words, or the cold shoulder. If you could see the insecure part, or parts, of yourself, what would it/they look like? Look within yourself and ask to see this frightened little part. How old is it? Two years? Six years? Twenty years? What is he or she doing? Is she huddled in a corner? Is he wide-eyed and frozen in terror? Most of us have three standard responses to our own insecurities: We're unaware of them, we ignore them, or we reject them. What would you be like - and what would your life be like - if you gave this part of yourself what it needed? What would you and your life be like if you actually took the time to listen to the insecure part of yourself? Often we tend to give in to our insecurities and abandon whatever it is that's making us nervous. But this doesn't really help because, if we could really hear what our little three-year-old was saying, we'd know that he/she isn't really asking us to return the new computer to the store. If we actually allowed ourselves to listen to what this part of ourselves wants, we'd hear that what it wants and needs is support, groundedness, and a sense of internal solidity in tackling this task of which it's so afraid (i.e., setting up the new computer). And, of course everyone's level of insecurity is different. Some of us feel confident about most things and have much more of an ease in navigating the waters of life, while others feel pretty insecure in general and see life as a screaming ride through treacherous rapids rather than a slow trip down a lazy river. The reality is that we all have this part of ourselves, and learning to recognize and support it is something that can be helpful to each of us, no matter our level of insecurity.

The Earth is a sphere, spinning in space. Every twenty-four hours (give or take a few minutes), it completes a full circle and comes back to the point at which it started. Every twenty-four hours, our planet goes from day to night, from light to darkness, and then back again. This ability to rotate and return to a certain point over and over again is something that we can use to comfort ourselves when we feel insecure, shaken, and homeless. If you want to work with your insecurity further, try to notice the next time that you're feeling this way, whether it's in the next five minutes, five days, or five weeks. Having a sensitivity to ourselves in this way isn't always easy; for, as I mentioned earlier, our tendency is to let our insecurities get the upper hand and shut us down ("O.K., I give up! What's the return policy on this thing?!?"), to chastise ourselves for them ("What are you so nervous about? It's a *computer*, for goodness' sake, not a beheading!"), or to miss their presence altogether. But try to notice when you're feeling this way. Often we experience certain emotional or mental states in specific parts of our bodies, and insecurity is no exception. For example, you might feel a nervous fluttering or flapping in your midriff area, as though you're about to come apart at the seams. Or you might feel a heaviness in your abdomen, or a tight band around your head. Once you've located it, focus your attention in that place, and allow yourself to see a small image of the Earth spinning there. If you're not feeling the insecurity anywhere in your body, don't worry. Just pick a place and allow yourself to see the Earth spinning there. Watch the image of the Earth spin for a minute or two and then try to see or feel or hear what's happening. What effect, if any, is this having upon you? Are you starting to feel more expanded, for instance, and less worried? Are you feeling less nervous? Has the ground stopped shaking? Do you feel more capable of dealing with the situation in front of you - the situation which caused you to feel insecure in the first place?

Doing this exercise is something that can give you information about your own level of insecurity and how to deal with it. You may find, for example, that it has a centering effect upon you. Or you might simply find it annoying or ineffective, in which case there are other ways of helping yourself become more self-supportive by using the returning, cyclic rhythms of life on planet Earth. Performing certain activities at regular intervals throughout the day is something which can bring this cyclic quality into our lives. For instance, eating on a regular schedule can be a very supportive thing for many of us (not to mention vital to the process of losing weight and then maintaining it). As a healthcare practitioner, I'm always amazed at the number of clients who seem to be able to go on practically nothing all day ("I have a bagel in the morning, and then a regular dinner at night.") because they really don't feel hungry until they stop to rest. The problem here is that the body needs fuel more frequently than twice a day; and when faced with an empty fuel tank, it's forced to resort to a lot of creative, and potentially harmful, alternatives. Then there are those of us who have no regularity whatsoever in the way that they eat: one day, it may be every four or five hours, the next day it may be every twelve. The problem with this is that, after a period of time, the body doesn't know from one minute to the next whether it's going to be faced with feast or with famine and this starts to create a sense of insecurity on a purely physical level.

Eating on a regular basis can establish a foundation which allows us to feel more secure. And when we feel more secure, we're able to expand our idea of who we are and what we can do and be. Children who are nurtured, held, and fed when they need it are often more likely to venture outside their protective circle and try new things; they have a view of themselves - and of life - which tells them that there is something in the world that will always be there for them, supporting them, no matter what. Because the energy of the cycle, or circle, is strongest during late summer, it's the best time of year to see and feel the effects of regular, cyclical behavior and feel the way it reverberates through our lives. And because this is the time of year when the energy of support is at its peak, we have a lot of help in establishing new routines which allow us to take care of ourselves. But it's important to remember that seasons are part of a yearly cycle, and thus each season has an effect upon the rest of the year. Making changes in the way you nourish yourself now, during this season of nourishment and abundance, will have effects which are felt throughout the next ten to twelve months. Life often holds many, many challenges and surprises for us, and it's much easier to face them when we're well-nourished and well-fuelled than when our tank's constantly close to "empty" and our bodies are traumatized by never getting what they need when they need it.

Adjusting your sleeping pattern to fit the daily, or diurnal, cycle of darkness and light can also be helpful. In modern times, we have technology which allows us to have light whenever we need it. But, in terms of human evolution, this development is exceedingly new while the blueprint for our bodies is exceedingly old, and thus most of us do much better when our patterns of sleeping and wakefulness are more in sync with the rising and setting of the sun. In other words, when we go to sleep an hour or three before midnight and wake up somewhere around sunrise, most of us sleep more soundly and awaken feeling more refreshed. As anyone who's ever suffered from sleep deprivation or chronic sleep disturbances knows, it's hard to face the day - and even harder to have a positive outlook - when we don't get the refreshment and replenishment we need from sleep, and matching our own bodily cycle to that of the planet is often helpful in this regard. Of course, there are those who are able to fall asleep and get the kind of rest they need any time of the day or night, but these people tend to be the exceptions rather than the rule. Most of us find it much easier to abandon body, mind, spirit, and emotions to the replenishing waters of sleep when our own body clock matches that of our planet's. But it's important to remember that everyone is different, and that good health doesn't mean "being good". In other words, I'm not saying that, in order to "be healthy" one must eat follow the planetary cycle of darkness and light. Good health comes from allowing yourself to be your own healer and trying to do what healers do: Listen to yourself and try to give yourself what you need. Sometimes irregularity in certain parts of our lives is just as healing as regularity is. A sense of personal freedom is the cornerstone of good health and so it's important to tend freedom's flame and keep it burning. So, if staying up until all hours is necessary to your sense of freedom, then by all means allow yourself to do this. Good health is a kind of fluidity which allows you to respond to what you need when you need it. Good health does not mean forcing yourself to march lockstep into the future, chanting, "I'm being good. I'm being good. I'm being good."

And then there are other activities and non-activities which can help us feel more stable. Morning activities often set the physical and mental tone for the day. Some of us need a morning routine where the same things are done in approximately the same order every morning. This type of regular routine establishes a stable foundation for the rest of the day; and once we have a foundation which is stable, what we build upon that foundation has a much better chance of being sound and stable as well. But there are others who need to start their day with a period of unstructured activity. While some of us bound out of bed at the first light of dawn, bright of eye and clear of purpose, and some of us like to follow the well-worn groove of sameness, others need to get up and mill around and do whatever seems to pop into their minds: look out the window, have a drink of water, a cup of coffee, watch the news, water the plants, try to identify the birds at the bird feeder, and make a few calls. These people like to wade into the day whenever possible; diving into it doesn't work for them. They need time to get into their bodies and find that this period of unfocussed meandering centers them. (Interestingly enough, a period of unstructured activity - at any time of the day - is often a helpful springboard to creative endeavors; for, contrary to what most of us believe, creativity usually arises out of chaos, not out of structure.)

Allowing yourself to do things that you feel you're "not allowed" to do can also be a good way to let the three-year-old inside feel less insecure and better taken care of. Many of us feel, for example, that we're "not allowed" (usually by ourselves, if we're adults and we live in a free society) to voice our opinions. Because some of us are inherently communicative, just allowing ourselves to be who we are - that is, to put things into words and then let those words come out of our mouths - can go a long way toward making us feel more connected to our core and therefore more secure as people. Often, we don't let ourselves voice these opinions because we're afraid of how they will sound, or we're afraid that what we have to say will be too damaging. And, yes, it's usually counterproductive to give someone both barrels and leave them lying in the dust. But the reality of giving one's opinion is rarely like this. The reality of saying "That was the worst movie I've ever seen" or "I really hated it when you told me I was overbearing" hardly ever has the power to reduce someone to emotional rubble. We usually have an overblown idea of the power of our own opinions because we're not used to voicing them. We've kept them locked safely away in a closet and, like anything that's been locked away in the dark for a long time, they've started to take on a lot more power than they actually have - the Power of the Unknown. And so, instead of seeing them for what they are

- views which may or may not be in agreement with the views of others - we start to see them as lethal weapons of mass destruction or something behind a door marked "Danger! High Voltage!". The reality is that everyone has opinions, and that our opinions are just as important - i.e., neither less nor more important - than everyone else's.

Mother Earth is there for us all the time, supporting us. If you need a direct experience of this, go outside and stand on her. When we press down on the breast of mother Earth, she presses back with equal force - or we'd fall through. The Earth is a small blue speck traveling through the darkness of space. There is beauty and poetry in this image, but there's loneliness and terror, too. So let yourself remember that the Earth, our home, our planet, our mother, is a solid thing made of rock and soil. And every twenty-four hours, she comes back to the exact same point she left twenty-four hours earlier, ready for another day, ready for another trip, ready for another twirl around her axis. So go outside and stand on the Earth, feel her support, and know that it's something which is always there for us. ♪♪

❦ The Bigger Picture ❦

The energy of late summer is a decidedly nonlinear one. It's the energy of the circle, the energy of a form which has no beginning and no end and which is going nowhere.

Often at the beginning of a new healing regimen, we try to be very disciplined and committed to our new venture and to our new image of ourselves. Perhaps, for example, we've decided that we're never, ever, ever going to eat any more refined sugar. And, after excluding it from our diet, we find that we honestly feel better and that our energy level is more constant; and this serves to bolster our conviction that refined sugar is evil and must never again pass our lips. But what do we do with the "old" image of ourselves? What do we do with the part of ourselves that really likes those Hershey bars and those cupcakes in the little cellophane wrappers? What do we do with the part of ourselves that still wants to eat something which our new, improved, and ultra-enlightened self considers to be nutritionally toxic? Most of us react to this dilemma by trying to distance ourselves from the mistaken, uninformed, and misbegotten part of ourselves. And we do this in the interest of going forward, in the interest of neatness.

Neatness is something which we human beings value, and rightly so, for neatness allows us to get things done. Neatness presupposes a landscape where everything is tidied up, where all the corners are squared and everything is put away into its little niche; all the mess is gone, resolved into cabinets which are organized and into drawers which are closed. Nothing is left unfinished, everything has been put into its place and remains there. Everything which is useless or redundant has been weeded out and thrown away, and nothing which is contradictory to the purpose at hand is allowed to remain. But the problem here is that neatness is not an energy which is compatible with healing. For healing is something which asks us to expand our idea of who we are and to approach ourselves with acceptance, and so it's a process of addition, not a process of subtraction. Thus, a healing approach to the self would be one which allows us to make room for both of these aspects: the part which rejoices at the thought of Hostess Ho-Ho's and the part which flinches at the thought of them. This ability to accept both parts of ourselves is something which takes us down the road toward healing, while its opposite - the inability to have an acceptance of any part of ourselves - takes us in the reverse direction, toward illness and pain.

Late summer is the time of year when the energy of abundance reigns supreme. It's the time of year when we can most clearly see that what the universe offers us is a feast, a cornucopia of plenty. As human beings we feel that who we are is limited by the boundary of our bodies; and so we tend to see life, not in terms of abundance, but in terms of limitation. The human consciousness, therefore, resonates more easily with the perception that life is limitation, a patchwork of unmet needs rather than a well-stocked refrigerator which is never empty. The aim of healing is to acknowledge the existence of both the limitless abundance of the universe, the ongoing and never-ending banquet, and the orphan part of ourselves which, out in the cold with its nose pressed up against the glass, has no idea how to open the door and join the feast. Neatness would dictate relegating this part of ourselves - the part that identifies with deprivation - to the garbage heap. However, compassion and acceptance, the cornerstones of healing, suggest that we include the orphan part of ourselves in the mix and that we all go forward together, no matter how unwieldy and messy this makes life seem. Neatness says that life is a gift, perfectly wrapped with paper creased to knife-edge perfection and a bow which is perfectly tied and properly attached to the box. Healing says that, yes, life *can* feel like a gift and that, yes, everything can go into the box together; but the fit will be imperfect, there will probably be some bulges, and the bow might not stay on because of all the commotion inside. So, during this season of feasting and plenty, allow yourself to embrace both the lack of order and the lack of uniformity which healing and expansion can bring. Life is a journey, not an endpoint. It's something which, like the process of healing, is ever-changing and not easily forced into a box. During these gentle, pale yellow days of late summer, allow yourself to embrace the process of life; allow yourself to participate in it and to welcome the messiness that abundance, acceptance, and compassion can bring us.

⚘The Body

The energy of each season is unique, and so each season has a unique and specific relationship to the body. For example, the incisive energy of autumn urges us to cleanse the body by letting go of what no longer serves us, while the quiet energy of winter asks us to rest and replenish our physical being. But the energy of late summer is the energy of the flesh; its voluptuous, sensual nature asks us to focus on the body itself, its needs and its pleasures. Here, then, are some ideas on how to take care of this aspect of our being.

Use It The body is the house of the mind, the emotions, and the spirit; but the body itself has its own reality, and that reality is grounded firmly in the physical. Thus, the body not only likes to be used, it actually needs this in order to stay healthy. For instance, when we pick up a child or do a headstand or lift weights, our bodies reward us by becoming stronger and healthier. How does using our bodies benefit them? Well, when we use our muscles, for example, they contract and this puts pressure on the corresponding bones. The bones then respond by laying down more bone tissue and, together with enough calcium in the diet, the result is that they become thicker and, consequently, stronger. In this way, using our muscles keeps our bones strong. When we do aerobic exercise - that is, exercise which elevates our heart rate - our bodies reward us for exercising our heart muscle and our lungs with increased energy, stamina, muscle tone, and heart health. Even vaginal thinning and friability - that is, the tendency to tear - in menopausal and post-menopausal women can be helped by using this area of sensuality and pleasure on a more regular basis.

So during this season of the body and its needs, take some time to look at how much - and how often - you use it. First of all, are you using your muscles enough? Do you get some kind of regular aerobic exercise, such as walking, swimming, running, cycling, etc.? This is the season of mother and mothering, and I don't want to sound as though I'm nagging you (although most of us would admit that nagging is usually done because the nagger cares very deeply for and is concerned about the naggee), but this is very important to long-term health. And it doesn't have to be strenuous aerobic exercise, though this is beneficial for many; it just has to be a moderate amount of exercise (twenty to forty minutes) at a slow to moderate pace on a regular basis. Three to four times a week is probably best for most of us, but if you can only manage two times a week, that is much, much better than no times a week. If, however, you're unable to exercise due to physical illness or limitations, try to introduce some physical activity into your life in some way. For example, you may have an illness which doesn't allow you to walk more than a few steps at a time, or you may be someone who is wheelchair-bound, yet there still may be some type of sustained activity which is possible for you. You may be able to do aerobic exercise with your arms; or your may still be able to use your legs if you're sitting down while doing it. It may be possible to find programs such as adapted aquatics or adapted physical education in your area. Your physician or physical therapist may be able to help you decide upon and locate an exercise plan. One client who was unable to sit on her stationary bicycle because of problems with balance told me that she had found that she could sit on the couch and pedal from there. This of course meant that she had to pedal much more slowly, and, because of her severe health problems, she could only last three to ten minutes at a time; but it was exercise and, again, some exercise is much, much, much better than none.

Secondly, are you exercising your bones regularly? The above-mentioned forms of aerobic exercise are helpful in maintaining bone thickness and strength, but they may need to be supplemented by lifting weights or by other exercises such as push-ups and chin-ups (or attempted chin-ups, as the case may be; don't let the fact that you can't do a chin-up deter you from getting and using a chin-up bar. Even if you can only lift yourself a measly two inches, you're still benefitting your muscles and your bones. And if you persist, you'll get better at it.) or floor exercises for the lower body. Another form of exercise which benefits the bones is yoga.[2] We usually tend to think of yoga as being a form of stretching to increase flexibility; but yoga has the potential to do much, much more. Many of the postures in the practice of yoga are very effective in "exercising" and strengthening the bones: Headstand, Shoulder stand, Down-facing Dog, Frog, just to name a few. (The practice of yoga also allows us to work with our energy systems in a very direct way; and many of the postures allow us to massage, and thus increase the health of, our internal organs.)

Third of all, and on a more delicate note: It's important for most of us - and perhaps all of us, though I hesitate to generalize because we're all so unique - to use our genitalia on a regular basis. It may seem ridiculous or embarrassing to some that I find it necessary to mention this; but everyone has a unique and special relationship to his or her own sexuality. And even though we live in a

---

[2] There are many different types of yoga. I am referring to the forms of yoga which use *asanas*, or postures, in order to tone and build the health of the body as well as the rest of our beings.

culture suffused with sex, sex, and more sex, sharing our sexual energy with another human being isn't on everyone's "to do" list. But in many ways, the health of these tissues depends upon their use. As I mentioned earlier, menopausal and post-menopausal women may experience thinning of the vaginal tissues; and often the very thing that helps to remedy this thinning is the stimulation - i.e., use - of this area. On the opposite side of the gender fence, the prostate (a walnut-sized gland that sits right below the bladder) is often kept in good health by having regular ejaculations. ♪

Listen to it. The body has many needs, and these needs are often very different from, and in direct conflict with, the needs of the rest of our being. How often have you turned a deaf ear to the body as it called out for something - a trip to the bathroom to empty a full bladder or a drink of water, for instance - because you were in the midst of something and couldn't be bothered? I'm not suggesting that we become a slave to our physical needs; I'm just asking you to give the body the consideration that it needs - and the consideration which it deserves. For our bodies, as annoying or embarrassing as they may be to us at times, do so much for us, and they do it all the time, even when we're not looking. For instance, right now there are several vital processes going on inside of each of us that are involuntary - that is, not under the control of our conscious minds. The process of digestion is one of these. The digestive tract is basically a tube that starts at one end of the body and ends at the other. Food is put into the mouth and then pushed through the tube by something called peristalsis. Peristalsis is a very fascinating thing. It's a unique type of wavelike contraction made possible by the action of a specific kind of muscle tissue called smooth muscle tissue. Unlike skeletal muscle tissue, which is only found attached to the bones and whose sole responsibility is moving them around, smooth muscle tissue is found in the walls of our organs (the uterus, urinary bladder and ureters, blood vessels, and respiratory passages). Skeletal muscle tissue is voluntary, or under our conscious control, while smooth muscle tissue isn't (which, of course, means that, once again, our bodies are doing things for us without our having to ask). Furthermore, skeletal muscle tissue can only be stimulated to contract by the nervous system, while smooth muscle tissue can be stimulated by neurotransmitters, hormones, or, in a feat of incredible mastery which has left physiologists shaking their heads in wonder, themselves. So the next time you get upset with your body because it has let you down in some way, think about the layer of smooth muscle tissue in your digestive tract working quietly away, making it possible for you to break down foodstuffs, extract and absorb nutrients, and send waste products to the large intestine to be eliminated - and all without being asked to do so.

We often find it hard to fill our physical needs because we're so used to ignoring the signals which tell us that we're hungry, thirsty, tired, uncomfortable, or in pain until we've gotten to the point of no return. Late summer is the time of year when the energy of needs and neediness is the strongest, and thus it's a time when the voices of our own needs are much louder and easier to hear. Take some time during the next week or so and make it a point to be more aware of what's going on with your body. It's difficult, or even devastating, when we have emotional, spiritual, or mental needs which are not being filled or acknowledged, and the same holds true for that other aspect of our being, the physical aspect. The energy of mother and mothering is the energy of someone extending his or her awareness outward toward another in order to ascertain what that other person needs; and cultivating an ability to be a mother to your own body will go a long way toward increasing your physical health, your physical well-being, and your sense of security on a physical level. Denying one's own physical needs can, over time, create a reality for the body which says that life is a barren and parched field where deprivation, pain, and discomfort prevail. Cultivating the ability to be a mother to your own body can go a long way toward increasing your sense of security on other levels as well. For, as any infant or small child would tell you if he or she could, being hungry, thirsty, tired, in pain or discomfort and being dependent upon someone who doesn't hear you is very destructive to one's sense of well-being. ♪

Nourish it. One of the problems in figuring out what to eat is that there is essentially no diet which is good for everyone. Some of us do much better on a vegetarian diet with little protein - that is, a diet high in complex carbohydrates - while others need a diet higher in protein and lower in complex carbohydrates. A small, yet significant, number of us can tolerate a certain amount of animal fat in our diet, while most of us can't handle this at all. Many of us do very well with fruits, while others can't tolerate the acidity and the sugars. Another problem is that many of us don't trust ourselves to make sane, intelligent decisions on how to nourish ourselves with food. Add to this the fact that the views of the alternative and western medical establishments, as well as those of the scientific community, change constantly and often contradict each other, as well as the fact that our air and water are polluted and our soil is losing its fertility, and you could just start screaming and never stop. How can you figure out what to eat? Allow me to offer some ideas:

❦*Listen to yourself.* The issue of what to feed ourselves is often clouded by the idea of what a nourishing diet "should" be. A further complication is that the body, the mind, the spirit, and the emotions very often have different needs. The body may be in need of some extra calcium and B-vitamins and so may be asking for broccoli or almonds, while the mind may want something to perk it up - coffee, for instance - while the emotions may be asking for something to comfort them, like toast and jelly or mashed potatoes. Start by asking yourself what you're hungry for. Try to put aside any preconceptions of what you 'should be' eating and listen to the answers that you get. Then notice what judgments come up. Do you automatically dismiss the part of yourself which is asking for something that you feel is 'unhealthy' - chocolate for example? (Most of us usually deal with this dilemma by eating it anyway and then feeling guilty afterward.) But chocolate is a rich source of potassium and antioxidants. It also has a certain amount of iron, and milk chocolate has a significant amount of calcium as well. Thus, as food for both body and emotions, chocolate offers us a lot. (The main problem with chocolate is that most of us tend to gravitate toward chocolate made with refined sugar. But very high quality, delicious chocolate made with less-refined and unrefined sweeteners is also easily available. Another problem with it is that chocolate also contains compounds which have an amphetamine-like effect upon us; so, unless you're using chocolate as a stimulant, it's best to approach your chocolate eating with moderation.) Next, try to figure out what the body itself is asking for. Some of us are very connected to our physical being and are able to distinguish its needs from those of the emotions, mind, and spirit. If you're not one of these people, however, it is possible, with practice, to cultivate this type of communication and awareness. So, after you've identified the judgments that you have, try to decide whether they're valid. If, for example, your body is asking for something which you know will give you a case of screaming heartburn, it's time to go on to the next menu selection.

❦*Notice how your body reacts to what you feed it.* What your body thinks about a certain food - that is, whether it likes that food and whether that particular food is beneficial to it - is reflected in how the digestive system responds. (It's good to bear in mind that sometimes the body's reactions can be altered by such things as severe stress or by drugs - prescription and otherwise - including alcohol, tobacco, and vast amounts of caffeine. In these cases, the answer we get may be that of the drug or the situation rather than that of the body itself.) So, simply put, how do you feel after eating something? Do you feel good? Do you feel a sense of ease in your digestive tract? Or do you feel too full even though you haven't eaten that much? Does your stomach feel irritated and uncomfortable? Are you starting to get heartburn? Do you feel bloated? Does it feel as though there's a pile of cement in your stomach? Do you feel like an anaconda - that, is you've just eaten a whole animal and now you need several days to work it through your system? Remember that digestion, like diet, is a completely individual process. There are no rules; a food which may flow easily through one person's stomach may cause a traffic jam in someone else's, so try to be open to hearing your body's reactions to food. If whole wheat bread gives you a stomach ache, it's not for you, no matter how rich in nutrients it is. And sometimes it's not a specific food which is giving us problems. Sometimes we're not digesting a certain food because of dehydration or because we're eating them at a certain time of day. And sometimes it's because of the way we're combining foods; for example, eating fruit together with meat or eating raw vegetables with raw fruit can give some of us a major case of the runs or the mother of all stomach aches.

❦ *A few guidelines.* We're all different and unique. Yet it's equally true that each of us is the same in certain respects. All human beings are warm-blooded, carbon-based animals breathing an atmosphere which is about 20% oxygen. The cells in our bodies - nerve, muscle, blood, and skin cells, for example - are identical to the nerve, muscle, blood, and skin cells of every other person on the planet (with the exception of those whose cells are modified by diseases such as sickle-cell anemia, for example); they all have the same structure and function, and they all have the same needs. I've come up with what I consider to be the five basic components to a nourishing diet and I'm offering them as starting points for those who feel they need some guidance. As you read them, bear in mind that, while these five fundamentals apply to most of us, they don't apply to all of us. Some of us need to be on restricted or modified diets because we have diseases of the kidney, heart, or gastrointestinal tract or because our bodies have been modified by surgery. And, as you read them, also bear in mind that, once again, you (together with your physician, if applicable) are the final authority.

First Fundamental: Vegetables. While fruits are sensual and wonderful sources of vitamins A and C, potassium, and magnesium, they're not absolutely necessary to everyone's health. It's possible to get vitamin C from baked potatoes, yams, tomatoes, broccoli, or sweet red peppers, and to get vitamin A from yellow and green vegetables. Vegetables are much denser in nutrients than fruits, which is good because there's a significant number of us whose bodies don't react favorably to fruit. But all vegetables are not alike; the dark leafy green vegetables are the most nutritious. They are: broccoli, chard, asparagus, beet greens, Brussel sprouts, bok choy, edible-pod peas, spinach, collards, dandelion greens, turnip greens, kale, and okra. These vegetables are the heroes of nutrition. Broccoli, for instance, has so many nutrients that it's almost ridiculous. It's loaded with calcium and iron and with vitamin A, the B vitamins, an appreciable amount of protein and vitamin C, and a ton of fiber, not to mention certain trace minerals. Try to have a least two servings (i.e., whatever a 'portion' means to you) of them a day. More than two is, of course, better for most of us. But if you're someone who has trouble including any dark leafy greens in your diet, one or two is much, much better than none.

🐦 *Second Fundamental: Oils.* Everyone needs to have 'good' oils in their diet. What's a 'good' oil? In the last decade or two, the prevailing opinion about fats and oils has changed many times, often fluctuating wildly from one extreme to another. We've gone from 'no fat' to 'low fat' to 'polyunsaturated fats such as corn or safflower oil are best' to what we have most recently, which is the idea that the monounsaturated fats, like olive and canola oil, are the "best" for us. There's a wealth of information out there about which oils to eat, and I think it worth your time to read up on the subject and form your own opinion. Most oils become rancid over time; while some oils like olive oil don't need to be refrigerated, others such as canola oil do. Fats and oils come from two basic sources: animal sources, such as butter, and plant sources, such as sesame, canola, and olive oil. Most - but certainly not all - of us can't really tolerate much, if any animal fat on a regular basis. But all of us - with some exceptions - need to eat good, fresh oils derived from plants sources every day. How much varies from person to person. If you're unsure, first check with your physician to see whether he or she feels you need to limit your intake of fats. Then, listen to yourself.

🐦 *Third Fundamental: Water.* We all need to drink enough water. Some of us have to limit our intake of fluids because of things like kidney or heart disease, but most of us don't. Check with your physician. "Enough" to me means at least two quarts of unpolluted water - not tea or broth or soda but just plain old water - each day for an adult human being. "Optimum" would be two-thirds an ounce of water per pound of body weight, or your weight multiplied by two and then this sum divided by three. Some of us need more water than others. For example, the more protein you ingest, the more water (and calcium!) you need. Dehydration is often difficult to detect; it's common to be dehydrated but not feel thirsty. In fact, dehydration can masquerade as seemingly unrelated things such as sleepiness, tiredness and even anxiety.

Recently, this idea that only water by itself counts as water has become controversial. Many now claim that any kind of liquid counts. But, personally and professionally, I disagree. I still believe that the concept "only water counts as water" holds true for the vast majority of human beings.

⚖ *Fourth Fundamental*: *Protein.* While carbohydrates such as grains and vegetables function mainly as sources of fuel, we need protein for the maintenance and repair of the body and for regulation of certain bodily processes. Everyone's need for protein is different. In general, children need more protein than adults because they're in the process of building their bodies. But as adults, the amount of protein which we need in our diet can vary greatly from person to person. Some of us need very little and do much better on a diet low in protein, while some of us need quite a bit and really can't function with less. For example, protein in the diet helps stabilize blood sugar levels, something which is vital to those of us with blood sugar issues. Like oils, protein comes from two sources: plant and animal. The protein in most plant sources is accompanied by a high concentration of carbohydrates, while the carbohydrate content in animal tissue is negligible. So, if you're someone who needs to eat a lot of protein while keeping your intake of carbohydrates to a minimum (e.g., someone who is hypoglycemic), you may need to turn to animal sources for the protein that you need. Eggs are a rich source of protein with a protein to carbohydrate ratio of about twelve grams of protein to one of carbohydrate; but if you're someone who has trouble digesting animal fat, or if you're someone who needs to cut down or eliminate it from your diet, try eating just the whites. An omelet made with egg whites can be very satisfying, especially when it's cooked in a fruity olive oil. And, of course, you don't have to be a purist; you can - health permitting - include a small amount of the yolk for the richness of taste and the added nutrients (among them, vitamins A and E, pantothenic acid, folacin, riboflavin, and thiamin). Some of us can tolerate, and may even need, beef on a regular basis, while for others this would be cardiovascular or digestive suicide. Often those who benefit from eating beef are those who approach life in a mental way; these people tend to live in their minds and beef has a grounding effect upon them which allows them to connect to their bodies. Some of us do very well on lighter proteins such as fish and fowl, but can't digest beef. Once again, listen to yourself. And if you need to eat animal protein but feel that you can't because of the way that animals are raised and slaughtered, it's becoming easier to find eggs from free-range chickens and beef and poultry which are raised with more consciousness for the animals' welfare. And then there's always fish.

With respect to plant sources, nuts and seeds are a rich source of protein. Almonds, pistachios, and walnuts have a one-to-one ratio of protein to carbohydrate. Pine nuts have a ratio which is close to three grams of protein to one of carbohydrate. (But pine nuts also contain goitrogens: substances which prevent the use of iodine, thereby affecting thyroid function. Other goitrogens are cabbage, turnips, peanuts, mustard, millet, and soy. But don't despair: Cooking inactivates goitrogens. Plus, goitrogens are not a problem for everyone.) Pumpkin seeds have a ratio of about two grams of protein to one gram of carbohydrates, and sesame seeds have a ratio which is about one to one. Peanuts are actually a legume like beans and lentils, and they have a one to one ratio of protein to carbohydrate. But most legumes have a ratio which hovers around one gram of protein to three grams of carbohydrate, with the exception of soybeans and tofu, which weigh in with a ratio of about one to one. The ratio in whole grains is much lower, ranging anywhere from one to twenty, to one to five - good news for the significant number of us who need to eat a diet low in protein. One caveat about nuts that grow on trees (like almonds, pistachios, etc. Peanuts - which are actually, again, legumes like beans - grow on vines.) is that many people have problems digesting and/or assimilating them. So, again, listen to what your body's telling you.

All fruits and vegetables also contain a certain amount of protein. The dark leafy green vegetables have the highest concentration. Broccoli, Brussel sprouts, and spinach, for example, have a ratio of about one gram of protein to one gram of carbohydrate, while chard, collard greens, beet greens, and kale have a ratio of about one gram of protein to two or three grams of carbohydrate. The concentration of protein in fruits is much lower. Strawberries, for example, have a ratio of about one to ten; honeydew melon, one to twenty-two; bananas, one to twenty-six; and blackberries, one to eighteen. Again, this is good news for those of us who need to have a diet low in protein and high in complex carbohydrates such as grains, beans, fruits, and vegetables. Thus, on the protein continuum, meat (i.e., any animal flesh) is at one end with whole grains and fruits at the other end. High-protein nuts, seeds, and vegetables are more or less in the middle, with the rest of the vegetables somewhere between them and the whole grains and fruits.

❦*Pay attention to time of day.* According to Chinese medicine, the time of day when our stomachs have the most energy - "stomach time" - is from 7:00 a.m. to 9:00 a.m. standard time (8:00 to 10:00 a.m. daylight savings time). Twelve hours later, between 7:00 and

9:00 p.m. standard time (8:00 to 10:00 p.m. daylight savings time) is "stomach low time", the time when our stomach energy is at its lowest ebb. In Chinese medicine, the stomach is one of the pillars of the digestive process, and so these two windows of time have two very important implications: The first of these is that our digestive tracts will have the greatest ability to handle whatever we give them during stomach time and the least ability to handle what we give them during stomach low time. In plainer English, it's best not to challenge our digestive tracts during stomach low time when our stomach energy is at its lowest ebb. This may not be the time, for instance, to eat vegetables or a huge, heavy meal because our digestive tracts just aren't up to the task at that time of day. The second implication is that, if we don't put something in our stomachs - i.e., food - during stomach time, we may very well find ourselves ravenously hungry twelve hours later. Thus, even though many of us don't have much of an appetite this early in the morning, it's a good idea to eat something anyway. And it doesn't have to be traditional breakfast fare. It can be something simple, such as a handful of almonds, a piece of turkey, a salad, yogurt, or leftover pizza. And liquids such as a glass of milk (cow's, soy, almond, or rice) or some diluted fruit juice are just fine if you can't deal with solids this early in the day. Even ice cream or frozen yogurt will work if that's all that your stomach will accept.

❦*Get a little sun.* Yes, it might be surprising to find the issue of sunshine under the heading of nourishment. But it's not an error. Within the last decade or so, research has begun to show how vitally important the hormone known as Vitamin D is to the entirety of who we are. Hormones (from a Greek word meaning "to set in motion") are regulatory substances; and if you think about the fact that we evolved in the sun, you can see how important being in the sun is to health. Living in the northern half of the United States, for example, makes us much, much more likely to get diseases such as multiple sclerosis. Taking supplements can be helpful, especially for those of us who live in Oregon or Maine, for instance, and have dark skin. But research is also showing that supplements can't do it alone, that there's no substitute for sunshine because the Vitamin D that our bodies make from the sun has a much longer half-life than the Vitamin D we ingest from supplements or from foods. Plus, there are other benefits from being in the sun: Sun baths set our circadian rhythm and regulate our sleep. Other necessary compounds such as photo-isomers are made in the skin. Being in the sun helps our mood.

There, of course, are some of us who cannot tolerate sunshine for medical reasons and therefore should never expose their skin to the sun. I urge you to consult with your doctor. And do some reading. At least one prominent researcher claims that, while sun exposure can lead to non-melanoma skin cancer, it does not lead to melanoma and in fact low Vitamin D makes melanoma more likely. The five external things we need are food, air, water, sunshine and love. So consult your physician. And, then, if you get the go-ahead, nourish your body with a little sunshine.[3]

❦ *Maximize calories.* Many of us tend to think about minimizing the damage to our waistlines rather than maximizing the nutritional value of what we eat. But it's very important to do so. Nutritionally speaking, a high percentage of what's offered to us in grocery stores and restaurants have taste and very little else to offer us. Frozen and canned vegetables and fruits are, with some notable exceptions, much lower in nutritional value than their fresh counterparts. Refined foods, such as white rice and bread made from white flour, are mostly empty calories, and because they're so prevalent, many of us are actually malnourished. It's possible to take supplements, but whole foods offer nutrients to the body in a way that is much more user-friendly - that is, presented to the body in a way that it understands - than supplements. But it's not just nutrients that are missing from refined foods; it's life force as well. For the more something is processed, the less energy or life force it has. This is one of the reasons that produce which is just-picked tastes so much better than produce which was picked yesterday or last week. Yes, certain biochemical changes start to take place the moment something is plucked off the vine or the tree, and this influences taste as well. But we beings of energy have a sensitivity, whether acknowledged or unacknowledged, to the energy around us and to the

---

[3] You can find detailed information on how and when to get sensible sun exposure in *The Vitamin D Solution: a 3-Step Strategy to Cure Our Most Common Health Problem* by Michael F. Holick, M.D., a physician and Vitamin D researcher.

energy that we bring into ourselves. And whole foods are a richer source of life force than processed foods. Again, I'm not advocating fanaticism or wild-eyed devotion to whole foods which makes you froth at the mouth at the mention of white sugar or white rice. It's possible to have these things in your life. I'm just asking you to take a look at your diet to see whether there's room for improvement in the nutrition department. So think about nutrition when you're deciding what to eat. Think about nourishing yourself.

♥ *Eat as cleanly as you can.* There may be no scientific evidence to support the idea that eating unsprayed or organically grown produce and meat from animals which are raised without hormones and antibiotics results in better health, but I personally just feel better eating this way whenever possible. Again, I can invoke the Caveperson Factor and wonder whether exposing ourselves to things such as herbicides, pesticides, and hormones is something which, over time, could very well have a negative effect upon us. There seems to be so much that we don't yet know about how these chemical compounds affect us. For instance, many dairy farmers in the U.S. give their cows recombinant bovine growth hormone (rBGH) in order to increase their milk production; and it's unknown how much of this actually gets into the milk and what effect, if any, it has upon us. All milk contains bovine growth hormone, or bovine somatotrophin, but recombinant bovine growth hormone is synthetically produced and injected into cows for the purpose of increasing their milk production. It's possible, at least in some places, to find milk from cows raised without it; and there's at least one nationally-known brand of ice cream and frozen yogurt which makes a point of using milk from cows who have not been given rBGH. ♪

Water it. The issue of drinking enough water bears repeating and even nagging. What I've found in my years as a healer is that a large - no, let me rephrase that to say a massive - number of us just don't drink enough water. And some of us don't drink any water. When clients tell me that their daily intake of water is zero, I tend to stare in disbelief and wonder aloud how they can still be breathing. Yet, years ago, I was in the same boat. The reality is that the body needs moisture in the form of water. Teas, coffee, and juices have their place, but all adults in good health need to give their bodies at least two quarts of unpolluted water - and that means water by itself, naked, and alone - every day. Children, of course, need water too. The rule of thumb is half an ounce of water per pound of body weight; or your weight divided by two.

The body needs a certain amount of water in order to carry out all that it has to do, from digestion to filtration. The kidneys and the bladder, as well as the circulatory system and the lungs, depend upon adequate moisture to function properly - and to function well over time. The skin needs water to stay healthy and supple. And, of course, water is vital to digestion; for, as anyone who's tended a compost pile knows, adequate moisture is necessary for decomposition. Since the first part of the digestive process is a type of decomposition, many problems can ensue if we're not properly hydrated, from indigestion to constipation to abdominal pain. Being properly hydrated is also important to the sinuses. From an energy standpoint, the sinuses are part of the digestive process because they're responsible for taking things in. Thus, sinus headaches and congestion can often be the result of not drinking the water that our bodies need. Finally, drinking enough water is of utmost importance to menstruating women, for dehydration can be a single, or contributing, cause of menstrual cramps.

And that's just in the short term. In the long term, it's very hard on the body to operate without enough water. Think of our poor little bodies, trying to grind along, year after year without the moisture that they need. The energy of water is the energy of refreshment, replenishment, and lubrication. It's the energy of flow. And in a very specific way, it's the energy of having enough resources. Think of the effect of being deprived of this energy of flow, this energy of lubrication, replenishment, refreshment, and the resources you need to get the job done - and to be deprived of this day after day, year after year after year. Let's face it. Anything - human body, lawnmower, or car engine - which relies upon lubrication for optimum performance will break down more often and fall apart much more quickly when deprived of this lubricant.

If you have trouble stomaching water, here are a few suggestions:

(1) Try it at a different temperature. If room-temperature water makes you gag, try it iced or very cold. If ice water doesn't agree with you, try it at room temperature. Or try drinking hot water. In other words, heat water as you would for tea but don't put anything in it. Drinking hot water can be helpful in opening up the nasal passages; it can also feel very soothing to the stomach, digestive tract, and even to the mind.

(2) If you need to drink bottled water, which many of us do because our local water is polluted, you may need to try different kinds of bottled water until you find one that you like. My experience has been that there's a vast difference in taste, and acidity, from one company to the next.

(3) Keep track of how much you're drinking. A good way to do this is to fill up a container or two in the morning with the amount you need to drink that day and then try to polish it off by the end of the day. And if you need an extra incentive, buy yourself something beautiful, such as a cut glass carafe or two; if this helps you drink the water you need, it will be money well-spent.

(4) If you drink coffee, try to drink at least a third to a half of your daily water before you have your first cup. Coffee tends to kill our thirst, and this makes drinking water very unattractive to us. And because coffee acts as a diuretic (that is, it promotes urination) we're dehydrating ourselves even more when we drink it. And those of us who drink coffee need to drink even more water in order to compensate for this loss of moisture.

(5) If drinking two or more quarts of water on a daily basis just seems too overwhelming to you, start small. Begin with the amount of water which seems the most manageable to you, and then, over the next few weeks, increase that amount. Clients who were new to the water habit and which took this stepwise approach to increasing their water intake usually tell me later that (a) it wasn't as hard as they had imagined to work up to two quarts a day; and that (b) after changing their drinking habits, they'd found that they'd developed a thirst for water which they were now able to recognize.

(6) Thirst from dehydration can masquerade as hunger; so, if you find yourself ravenously hungry and unable to satisfy your appetite, try drinking some water - or a lot of it - and see whether that takes care of your hunger.

(7) Finally, some of us just can't seem to stomach water at all; sometimes this is due to a disease process or to the effect of drugs. If this applies to you and you truly can't deal with water in its naked state, try adding fruit juice to your water and see whether this helps. Start with one tablespoon per quart, and then, if necessary, increase the amount of fruit juice in increments of a tablespoon until you've got something which is palatable to you. In my opinion, only water by itself has the desired effect upon the body, so it's best to start small and to proceed slowly. Some fruit juice suggestions are: pear or apricot nectar, organic grape juice, black cherry juice, or freshly-squeezed lime or orange juice. Try to find these juices sweetened with unrefined sweeteners (usually white grape juice) rather than with refined sugar. The organic grape juice in particular has an incredibly wonderful taste, and is nothing like its refined-sugar-sweetened counterpart. Pear nectar and apricot nectar tend to be less acidic, while citrus juices and grape juice tend to be more acidic. I've found that the very few clients who can't drink water without feeling sick are those whose stomach acidity has been influenced by long-term use of a combination of tobacco and caffeine or by certain medications. The stomach is an interesting little organ. It's naturally quite acidic because the hydrochloric acid which it secretes keeps its pH at 0.8 to 3.0. (To give you a yardstick, a neutral pH is 7.0; the pH of lemon juice is 2.5; of coffee, 5.0; of saliva, 6.3 to 7.3; and that of distilled water is 7.0.) The stomach needs to be this acidic in order to do its job, and when that acidity is changed, digestive problems can result. In fact, the stomach secretions are so acidic that the stomach itself needs to be protected from its own acidity; it does this with a specially-constructed lining covered in a layer of especially thick and sticky mucus. ⚘

Try to figure out what it needs when it's in pain and give that to it. Pain is something which usually gets our attention because it hurts and we don't like it. Chronic pain can be debilitating and, in the very long term, quite wearing on the spirit. This is because pain tends to make us feel isolated from everything and everyone around us, and this sense of isolation goes a long way toward increasing our suffering. In the twenty-first century, we have over-the-counter and prescription medications for pain, and very often these can be lifesavers. But pain is usually the symptom, the warning light which tells us that something is wrong; and so getting rid of the pain does nothing to treat the underlying problem which is causing the pain. Here are some things we can do for ourselves which can also be quite effective in addition to, or instead of, taking pain medication.

❧ *Check your diet.* For those of us who have either osteoarthritis or rheumatoid arthritis, eliminating certain foods can help decrease our level of pain. These foods include members of the nightshade family (white and russet potatoes, tomatoes, peppers, chilis, and eggplants) and citrus fruits and juices (lemons, limes, oranges, tangerines, grapefruits, tangelos). Even if you haven't been diagnosed with an arthritic condition, if you're in pain, it may be worth your time to try a little experiment: Eliminate these things from your diet for two or three days. You may notice a decrease in your pain level after you've stopped eating them; or you may notice that your level of pain has increased after you've added them back into your diet. (If you do add them back in, reintroduce them one at a time; this way, you'll be able to identify the culprit(s).) Either way, you'll have some valuable information about how your body responds to these foods. I know that it's often difficult to follow a diet which doesn't include nightshade or citrus, since most of the cuisine of the U.S. seems to be based upon tomatoes, potatoes, peppers, and citrus, but you may find that the tradeoff between less pain and a more restricted diet is a worthwhile one. And you don't have to be a purist. You may decide that you're going to have French fries for dinner every once in a while even though you know it will make your hands ache the next day, but at least you'll know what's making your body hurt. Having awareness increases our level of clarity, and the greater our clarity, the less our suffering.

There's also a condition known as "nervous bladder" or "interstitial cystitis" which mimics bacterial infections of the bladder but which is not caused by a bacterium. Some of the symptoms include frequency of urination with very little output and pain or discomfort in the bladder; and sometimes the urine has a very strong, foul odor. Often, your physician will have information on foods to stay away from, and these include aged proteins such as yogurt and cheese, and acidic foods such as citrus fruits and juices and red wine. Drinking enough water is of vast importance to decreasing, and even eradicating, the symptoms of interstitial cystitis. Caffeine, especially from coffee, can also increase the symptoms of discomfort and frequency, partly because coffee's acidic and partly because caffeine is a diuretic and depletes the body of water.

♈ *The menstrual cycle.* Menstruation can also be a pretty painful affair, as many of us know all too well. If you're someone who has painful periods, here are some things to think about.

(1) First of all, make sure you're drinking enough water. Water is a lubricant, and often menstrual cramping is at least partly due to dehydration. Diuretics are substances which allow us to reduce swelling, and water is actually the best diuretic, believe it or not. For, when the body is deprived of enough water, it tends to hold on to what it's got. This causes fluid to build up in the tissues, and swelling and bloating are the result. So the next time you experience cramping with menstruation, try drinking several glasses of water. Then increase your daily consumption to at least the recommended level: half an ounce of water per pound of body weight.

(2) It's also good to cut down or eliminate sources of caffeine during menstruation because of

caffeine's diuretic effect. The stimulant effect of caffeine is something which can also cause menstrual cramps to become more frequent and more intense. And caffeine tends to deplete us of iron, something we're losing anyway at this time, and calcium, the mineral which plays a huge role in muscle tension and nervous system functioning.

(3) Diet is important when we're menstruating. Because of the hormonal fluctuations in their bodies, menstruating women often notice that their digestive tracts are much more sensitive and finicky. Try to notice what types of things work for you. You might be surprised; fresh foods such as lettuce and steamed vegetables might be just the thing. Or you may find that you need extra protein during this time of month, for protein has a diuretic effect and can help with swelling and bloating. And try to listen to your cravings without becoming a slave to them. If, for instance, you crave something like chocolate, let yourself have some. Chocolate has an appreciable amount of iron and a plentiful supply of potassium, which we need during this time; and milk chocolate can offer us calcium. But try to keep in mind that chocolate also has some chemical components which have an amphetamine-like effect on us and thus too much (whatever that means for you) could very well be counterproductive.

(4) Make sure you have enough calcium in your diet. (See "Exercise" section below for ideas on calcium sources.) A lack of calcium can cause something known as premenstrual tension or PMT.

Premenstrual tension does not cause pain on the physical level, but it causes an enormous amount of emotional upheaval for both the menstruating woman and the unfortunate bystanders (usually her family), and this makes the pain more unbearable and harder to deal with. PMT is aptly named, for its main symptom is a kind of tension which feels as though one's nervous system is a rubber band which is being wound tighter and tighter until it finally reaches the breaking point. Women experiencing PMT are overly-reactive to stimuli, much more angry and combative than usual, and very, very easily frustrated. And when they reach the breaking point, there's usually a Vesuvius-like spewing of frustration and emotion that is so disruptive (and distasteful to the woman herself) that one client described her menstrual persona as "the bloodsucking alien". It's much easier to deal with the physical pain and discomfort of menstruation when your emotions aren't ricocheting off the walls and you hate yourself because you're biting everyone's head off.

(5) If you use tampons, try changing to all-cotton tampons which are additive-free and which are not whitened with chlorine bleach. This can often reduce or eliminate cramping. (Most "health food" or "natural food" stores or sections on your grocery store carry these.)

(6) Finally, it is said that, during menstruation, the door between the two worlds - the seen and the unseen - opens up. So, during this time of the month, try to take it easy. There's often a marked difference in the way that we feel during menstruation and the way that we feel during the rest of the month, so try to approach life in a way which acknowledges this. For example, we often feel weaker physically and more sensitive emotionally. Some of us experience heavy blood loss, which can take its toll on us. (Of course, if your blood loss is too heavy, please see your doctor right away.) And some of us can even have pain with our periods which ranges from annoying to debilitating. The menstrual cycle is another expression of the returning nature of the earth element. And, just as with any cycle, there's a period of waxing and a period of waning. So, when your time of the month comes, let yourself wane. Let yourself be more receptive and less active. Try to make the time and the space to give yourself over to this part of your monthly life which, for most women, spans thirty or forty years. This isn't easy for many of us who are busy with children, job, and home; and some of us just plain resent the disruption which menses can bring. But see what you can do. Look at your life and try to see where and how you can slow down, even if this just means sitting down more often. A woman's body is a lot like the Earth. It's round, it gives birth, it nourishes, and it has cycles. Try to see whether there's anything in this image which can help make your time of the month an easier one.

❦ *Headaches.* Because each of us has an energy system which is unique, some of us are prone to headaches and some are not. And some of us have suffered head or neck injuries which then make us more susceptible to pain in that area. I can't begin to address the subject of headaches in its entirety because headaches come in a variety of forms - sinus and tension headaches, to name two - and have a multiplicity of causes. However, there are three things which often play a role in all types of headaches as either causative or contributing factors, and so they're worth mentioning: **(1)** Dehydration. **(2)** Low blood-sugar. **(3)** Input overload. Thus, the next time you get a headache, check in with yourself to see whether any of these three apply to you and try to drink more water, eat something, or adjust the amount of input you're being subjected to. Unfortunately, migraines, that most terrible of headaches, seem to work according to different rules; and, once a migraine gets started, it's often impossible to stop it in its tracks but it is possible to lessen its severity or shorten its duration by eating something and/or drinking several glasses of water.

❦ *Make later life changes easier.* Pre-menopause, menopause and the kinds of changes that men go through as they near age 50 ('male menopause' to some) are not for sissies. Our energy systems are constantly changing as we go from infant to child to teenager to adult to older adult to, if we're lucky, elder. These are huge, deep changes in the cores of our beings, our energy systems, which are manifested physically, mentally, emotionally and on the spirit level. So it's good to do whatever we can to make it easier for ourselves.

Energetically, water is fluid. It lubricates It smooths the way. Think of a stream rushing down the side of a mountain. When it encounters a boulder, it doesn't freak out and run back uphill. It doesn't stop. It flows around the boulder, or over or under it. It takes the boulder in its stride. There's an acupuncture point, "Greater Mountain Stream". It's a water element point and when it's needled, it makes this ability to take things in stride, to go with the flow more available to that person. Drinking enough water at this point of our lives can be our "Greater Mountain Stream". For example, as we get closer to fifty, most of us have less energy to do things. In fact, one of the common symptoms of pre-menopause is periodic exhaustion. Proper hydration allows us to make more energy. Rest is important during pre-menopause, but we also have to get things done, and having enough - or more - energy with which to get things done makes our lives easier.

During this time of life, our connective tissue tightens and we're naturally a lot stiffer. Hydrating can help here as well. How? you may ask. Well, for one thing, not giving the stomach enough water to digest things makes it tighten up, kind of like a fist. When the stomach tightens, it pulls on the sheet of connective tissue that runs up the esophagus and attaches to the neck. Since our connective tissue is already tighter and less elastic at this stage of life, we feel it more and odds are good that we'll experience neck stiffness or pain. Or we may feel it in other parts of the body that are connected to the neck, such as the mid-back or low back.

Later in life, our hormone balance shifts. The reproductive hormones in women are designed to communicate with and influence the involuntary or smooth muscle tissue that lines the uterus and Fallopian tubes. But the entire digestive tract is also lined with this kind of muscle, which is why it's quite common for women to experience bowel irregularities right before menses. So, as our hormonal balance shifts in later life, we start to have more digestive issues - indigestion, gas, bloating. The first part of the digestive system is the stomach, which is in many ways like a compost heap because it's the place where the breakdown of foodstuffs is begun. As anyone who's ever intentionally or unintentionally composted anything knows, it doesn't happen without enough moisture. So helping the digestive tract do its job more easily - and better - by drinking enough water helps here as well.

❦ *Assess your coffee usage.* I love coffee. It's a wonderful, sensuous thing. As a drug, coffee has some very valid uses: for one thing, it tastes and smells wonderful and it's often a great, short-term antidepressant and pick-me-up. Recent [4] research shows that it may be a treatment for Alzheimer's Disease. Because it acts to constrict blood vessels, it can also be an effective nasal decongestant (though of course caffeine's ability to temporarily reduce the diameter of our blood vessels is also one of its dangers when looking at such things as heart health.) The caffeine in coffee can also boost athletic performance and relieve pain. And the caffeine in coffee also has the ability to raise our blood sugar with the result that we have more energy, at least in the short-term. Everyone's relationship to coffee is different: Some of us can tolerate coffee and some of us can't. And, as with other

---

[4] i.e., as of 2010

drugs, we tend to build up a tolerance to the caffeine in coffee, and then begin to need more and more of it to get the desired effect.

However, there are two faces to every coin, and the very properties which make coffee so wonderful can also cause us problems. Because of the way it affects the body, coffee prepares us much more for dealing with impending physical doom and mayhem than for day-to-day functioning and health. The caffeine in coffee turns on all the switches which allow us to face danger and defend our lives: it heightens our senses and our mental clarity, increases our energy level while decreasing our hunger and our thirst, and it decreases pain and empties our stomachs. In the land of coffee, there is no future; there is only a Now which needs defending, and every available physical and mental resource is geared toward this defense. Thus many of the effects of coffee make it hard, or even impossible, to be in touch with what's going on inside of us physically or emotionally. For one thing, coffee tends to get rid of our thirst so that, even though we may need to drink water, we don't feel thirsty and so we don't. Add to this the fact that coffee also increases urination, and you could end up becoming very dehydrated. And, like it or not, we need to drink enough water (those of us with kidney or heart disease need to be careful and follow our M.D.'s orders here), or we can start to experience such things as pain in the digestive tract, since an adequate amount of moisture is needed to break down and absorb foodstuffs and eliminate wastes, or pain in the bladder (especially if we're prone to the above "nervous bladder") or in the lower back. Coffee's ability to raise our metabolism and depress our appetite can often be helpful for those of us who need to lose weight, but not that great for those who need to eat regularly. For coffee's ability to prepare us for life-threatening situations by emptying the stomach tends to make the stomach respond more like a clenched fist than a receptacle for nutrients. So, drinking too much coffee or drinking it at the wrong time of day, can backfire: We don't eat enough when we need to and then find ourselves ravenously hungry later in the day and end up overeating. For some of us, this just represents a glitch in our diet plans; for others who have blood sugar problems (hypoglycemics and diabetics), it's much more serious.

Coffee increases our fire energy, getting us all fired up and feeling invincible. It also increases our physical performance. And the caffeine in coffee also has the ability to decrease pain, something which makes us love coffee even more. But pain can be an invaluable tool when trying to understand what's happening inside of us because it's often a signal that something is wrong. So, for instance, when we're in the land of coffee, we're less likely to get the message that we have a pulled muscle and more likely to do something which leads to further injury. And coffee can have direct and indirect effects upon the functioning of our nerves and muscles, for taken in large amounts (the definition of which varies from person to person), coffee depletes the body of calcium and potassium. Calcium, the most plentiful mineral in the body, is an essential ingredient in both muscle contraction and nerve impulse transmission. Potassium is one of the ions which, together with its partner sodium, creates the necessary chemical climate which allows nerve impulses to flow along nerve fibers. We may see the contraction of muscles and the flow of nerve impulses as single events, but they're not. They're actually the end result of a wonderfully-choreographed series of occurrences which must take place in a certain order and with very specific components; and calcium and potassium are two of these components. Another effect of the caffeine in coffee is that it makes it easier for nerve impulses to flow with less stimulation; thus, in plainer English, caffeine tends to give us a hair trigger, allowing us to explode much more easily and with less provocation. Too much coffee, as many of us have found out from unfortunate personal experience, can cause us to be jumpy, overly anxious, and to exhibit many of the personality traits of a cornered snake. (As a point of interest here, calcium deficiency is often the cause of what is known as premenstrual tension, the symptoms of which closely mimic those of being over-caffeinated. And not getting enough calcium in the diet can often be the cause of heart palpitations in women, especially those who are pre-menopausal and/or menopausal.) Finally, even though the caffeine in coffee is a very effective pain-reliever, it's also something which can aggravate pain which already exists. This is because caffeine acts to constrict blood vessels (something which also raises our blood pressure). When the blood vessels are constricted, the flow of blood to an area is reduced, producing the above-mentioned effect of worsening pain. Drinking coffee throughout the day acts to constrict the blood vessels for long periods of time and is more likely to have this effect.

❦ *Exercise.* Often when the body isn't getting the type of physical stress that it needs, it lets us know this by giving us a signal, and often that signal is pain. If you have pain which seems to be muscular in origin and it doesn't respond to stretching or resting it, try some weight-bearing exercise. For example, if you wake up from a good night's sleep with neck pain, and the neck pain doesn't get better with stretching, sometimes arm exercises with weights or push-ups will be effective in reducing or eliminating the pain. (Of course, listen to yourself. If you have pain, numbness, or tingling down a limb, for instance, or if the pain gets worse while you're exercising, stop and don't do anything else until you consult your physician.) And make sure you're getting enough calcium in your diet. Exercising your muscles also puts pressure on the bones; and, as I mentioned earlier, this is a trigger for the body to lay down new bone cells. But the body can't create new bone tissue without calcium. A calcium-rich diet can probably help lower your pain levels somewhat, but getting enough calcium is vitally important and completely indispensable when it comes to bone health. Brittle bones are bones which fracture easily. Women who are on the road to menopause, or those who have already arrived there, or teenage girls who aren't getting enough calcium or who are drinking caffeine or soft drinks (which, like high protein diets, deplete the body of calcium) are often risk for brittle bones; but anyone of any age or gender can develop brittle bones if they're not getting enough calcium and weight-bearing exercise. Today we have lots and lots of nutritional supplements available to us, but I feel that it's best to avoid taking non-plant-based supplements (including antacid tablets which are used as calcium supplements), and especially to avoid taking them over the long-term.

The reason for my bias is the Caveperson Factor: In order for our bodies to absorb the calcium they need from the digestive tract and to utilize it, the calcium has to be presented to our bodies in a form that they understand. The blueprint for the human body is thousands upon thousands of years old, while supplements have only been around for a few decades. Plants have also been around for millennia and the human body is therefore much more able to recognize and absorb the nutrients from plant sources, such as herbs and foods, than it is from supplements. Food sources of calcium are best: dark leafy greens (such as broccoli, chard, and spinach), almonds, salmon, and dairy products such as milk and yogurt, for instance. There are also foods which are used as herbs, such as nettle leaf, which are very high in calcium and present it to the body in a recognizable, easily digestible, and absorbable, form. Made into a tincture or infusion[5], nettle leaf is a wonderful, easily-absorbed source of calcium as well as a source of many other vitamins and minerals. And because it's a food, nettle leaf has no toxicity (though it's possible to be allergic to it, just as it's possible to be allergic to any food). Dandelion root is another food which can be used as an herb; it doesn't have as much calcium as nettle leaf, but it still has an

---

5 A tincture is made from soaking the herb in an alcohol base for several weeks. You can find them at "natural" food or "health" food stores. An infusion is simply a tea which has been brewed for a long time. The proportions are two handfuls (one ounce) of herb to a quart of boiling water. Steep six hours for leaves, eight hours for roots; strain, and drink one to two 8 oz cups a day.

appreciable amount as well as other nutrients. Nettle leaf has an energy which resonates with that of the earth element, while the energy of dandelion root is more in alignment with the wood element and the energy of springtime. Both nettle leaf and dandelion root are tonics for the body, and dandelion root is an especially good spring tonic. Dandelion root can also be taken as a tincture or an infusion. However, dandelion root also increases hydrochloric acid production in the stomach, and for some of us, this can mean an upset stomach or a stomach ache. If you notice any digestive distress, try cutting back to half of the dosage you were taking, or stopping altogether. Or, if you're taking the tincture, try switching to the infusion, since the tincture seems to do this more readily than the infusion does. If you're already taking the infusion, try infusing it for a much shorter period of time - 30 minutes to an hour.

❦*Cigarettes.* Smoking cigarettes is something which can also contribute to physical pain. One of the long-term effects of smoking tobacco is that it dries out the little pads between the vertebrae, the small bones of the spine. These spongy pads, which are called intervertebral discs, act to cushion the vertebrae from one another; they also absorb the shock to the vertebral column from regular daily activities such as walking, running, lifting, etc. In our youth, the discs are about 90% water, but this percentage decreases as we age; this gradual drying-out of the discs, when combined with weakening of the ligaments in the area, is something which makes our discs more prone to injuries in which part of the disc ends up protruding (a "slipped disc"). If the protruding portion presses upon nerve endings, it can cause pain in different parts of the body. Smoking cigarettes doesn't directly cause this injury to our discs; but it does tend to accelerate the natural ageing process which leads to this type of problem. Nicotine, the addictive ingredient in tobacco, can also act to constrict the blood vessels in the abdominal organs and cause tightness and consequent pain in different places in the body, such as the shoulders and neck.

And there's another aspect of cigarette smoking which can lead to pain. Tobacco is also a member of the nightshade family and breathing tobacco smoke is something which can be the cause of pain from osteoarthritis and rheumatoid arthritis, or it can worsen already-existing pain. This means that nonsmokers should avoid breathing secondhand cigarette smoke and that smokers should have their cigarettes outside so that they're not getting a double dose of it. Of course, from the standpoint of healing one's arthritis, the best thing would be to quit, but nicotine is quite addictive and often this is much easier said than done. And many of us like smoking and don't want to quit. Cigarette-smoking has become demonized in the past few years; and in some ways this is understandable, because the secondhand smoke affects the nonsmokers who are breathing it, and it does so in a very harmful way. But everyone needs, and deserves, compassion, and this includes those of us huddled over our cigarettes, furtively pulling smoke into our lungs and fouling the air. So, if you're a smoker and quitting isn't in your immediate future, give yourself a break and take care of yourself by smoking outside. And take care of others by

having your cigarettes where they won't be forced to
breathe what you're smoking. *⌀*

Accept it. Having a body allows us to do things which we
couldn't do without one: kiss someone, drive a car, get a
massage, eat food, run in place. But our bodies can also
limit us in certain ways. For instance, the mind is often able
to see how to do something in the blink of an eye, but it
usually takes the body a much longer time to get things
done. You may be able to understand exactly how to do a
pirouette in ballet class, for instance, long before your body
is able to execute one. Or you might be able to see very
clearly how to drive a car with a standard transmission; but
once you try to coordinate the gas, the clutch, and the stick
shift without stalling out or getting into an accident, it's
another story. Often this discrepancy between how the
mind sees things and how the body carries them out leads
to a lot of impatience with ourselves. After all, we tell
ourselves, It's simple! Can't you see how to do it? The
problem here is that the mind and the body operate
according to completely different rules. For example, the
mind doesn't have to develop the strength of certain muscle
groups, learn fine motor skills, or figure out how to
coordinate feet, hands and eyes in order to do things,
whereas the body does. And, compared to the mind, which
often operates on split-second timing, the body is on a
time-schedule which more closely resembles that of
continental drift.

    So take some time here and there during this season
of sensuality and plenty. Try to notice how you react to
your body when you feel it's limiting you, and then try to
cultivate an acceptance of it in all its crudeness and wonder.
Often as human beings, we tend to ricochet from one

extreme to the other when approaching our bodies: When we're trying to get things done, for example, we tend to see the body as the Only True Reality. When we're dealing with matters of the spirit, however, we tend to view the body as an annoying pet which is dirtying up the living room. Try to remember that it's the body's very crudeness, or earthiness, which allows us to enjoy the crunch of a carrot or the tartness of a glass of wine, the softness of a loved one's hand or the smoothness of the wind against our skin. Because of our physical needs, which often seem to embarrass us or get in the way of accomplishing things, and the ways in which our bodies seem to limit us, it can be very difficult to have an acceptance of this very animalistic part of ourselves. When dealing with the body, it's good to remember that healing is not a streamlined event in which everything fits neatly into its assigned space. Health and healing are not destinations at which we arrive and then remain forever. Health and healing are processes, not endpoints; they're not something that we can "get done" and then be done with. Health and healing are the processes of accepting who we are - and part of who we are is a body. The energy of the earth element is the energy of a basket, something which can hold a monkey wrench, a piece of fruit, and a sweater - things which are very different in both nature and function from each other. So during this time of the flesh, its demands, its challenges and puzzlements, try be like the basket which just accepts and doesn't judge. Try to cultivate an approach to yourself which can hold the unique realities of the body along with those of its companions: the mind, the spirit, and the emotions. Try to have a generosity toward this very precious vehicle, this amazingly intricate marvel which labors day after day and year after year to give us that which we hold so dear: a vantage point which allows us to glimpse the infinite from the standpoint of singularity. ❀ ❀ ❀

⚓ Gravity never sleeps. ⚓

Gravity never sleeps. The two compass points we use to navigate through life, time and space, exist together as a continuum, the warp and the weft of the fabric of space-time, the medium in which we float, raisins in the raisin bread of life, almonds in the universal candy bar, islands defining the shape of the sea which links them. But gravity ... gravity is the attraction, the pull of one object for another caused by the impression made by objects in the springy, flexible material of space-time. Anything that has mass, any object, has the ability to make this impression and change the shape of the space-time fabric around it, and in so doing, it opens up a channel, an invitation to other objects to fall toward it as effortlessly as water flows off a duck's back, as surely as leaves fall toward the soil, as naturally as a lover falls into the waiting arms of his beloved.

Planets have a huge enough gravitational pull that we stay stuck to its surface and things like the moon orbit us instead of flying out into space. But even a paperclip has the ability to deform space-time, to exert a gravitational pull and attract things to it. Even a paperclip or a butterfly or a mote of dust makes an impression and leaves its mark.

The universe curves. We see that now. Light, because it has weight, is bent by the curve of the space through which it travels. And, because it has weight, light responds to the pull of the physical, following the channel that objects open up because they are objects. The sun changes the shape of the space-time around it in such a way that it pulls planets millions and millions of miles from its center toward it and keeps them there, spinning and spinning, circling and circling it in orbit. The Earth curves, bending the fabric of space-time, and, stuck to her back, we fly at a thousand miles per hour while standing perfectly still through darkness that is full of light which falls toward us at 186,000 miles per second. And all because of attraction. All because of

curving. All because of gravity. The next time you doubt your
ability to perform magic, think of this.

❦ ❀ ❀ ❦

Bibliographic Resources

The foot:

Your Feet Don't Have to Hurt, Suzanne M. Levine, D.P.M., St. Martin's Press, New York, N.Y., First Edition, June, 2000.

The Complete Foot Book, Donald S. Pritt and Morton Walker, Avery Publishing Group, Inc., Garden City Park, N.Y., 1992.

The Foot and Ankle Sourcebook, M. David Tremaine, M.D. and Elias M. Awad, Ph.D., Lowell House Books, Los Angeles, 1995.

The high protein vegetables:

Laurel's Kitchen, Laurel Robertson, Carol Flinders and Brian Ruppenthal, Ten Speed Press, Berkeley, California, 1986.

Sunshine:

The Vitamin D Solution: a 3-Step Strategy to Cure Our Most Common Health Problem, Michael F. Holick, M.D., Hudson Street Press, New York, N.Y., 2010.

⇒ The Future ⇐

The Fifth Season is available as an ebook on Amazon. There is also a sound recording of portions of the book. Call me at 916.452-5995 or email me at *debbie@debbiejolly.com* if you are interested.

Debbie Jolly has been practicing classical acupuncture since 1986. She likes to have thoughts about things like fractals, quantum physics, movies, the energetics of politics and clothing. Her Desert Isle Pick Book is the dictionary. A graduate of the Master's of Acupuncture program of Tai-Sophia in Maryland (now MUIH), she lives and works in Sacramento, California, plays violin and co-writes original songs in a progressive trance-folk duo with her musical genius husband, Robert Jolly, and dabbles in playwriting, poetry, painting, photography and fashion. She is also making a film version of her play, "Is", which should be available for public consumption in the near(ish) future.

debbie@debbiejolly.com